input 2/17/23
DATE DUE

Common Cures for Common Ailments

Common

Albert Marchetti,M.D.

Cures for Common Ailments

 STEIN AND DAY/*Publishers*/New York

First published in 1979
Copyright © 1979 Albert Marchetti
All rights reserved
Designed by Ed Kaplin
Printed in the United States of America
Stein and Day/*Publishers*/Scarborough House
Briarcliff Manor, N.Y. 10510

Library of Congress Cataloging in Publication Data

Marchetti, Albert.
     Common cures for common ailments.

     Includes index.
     1. Medicine, Popular.   I.   Title.
RC81.M35   616   77-16114
ISBN 0-8128-2317-6

*To the better health of people everywhere
through self-awareness and personal control*

Acknowledgments:

Peter Miller
Sol Stein
Bonnie Miller
Albert E. Marchetti, M.D.
Alan Braunstein, M.D.
Wallace Exman
Elizabeth Spedale
John R. Cushing
Allan C. Watkins, J.D.

Contents

The author has compiled this guide to home remedies so that the reader will know that such remedies exist. The information herein provides the layman with a means of combating certain minor illnesses without the cost of going to the doctor.

The reader, however, should understand that the medications presented in this book are not a substitute for the thorough medical care and attention given by the highly trained and equipped doctor, assisted by a competent staff and the latest developments of medical science.

Should an illness persist or a condition become aggravated, the reader should immediately see a physician for further complete evaluation and possible treatment.

If an adverse reaction to any of the products mentioned in this book should occur, the medication should be discontinued at once and a doctor consulted immediately.

Foreword

One hundred percent of all teenagers suffer from acne and approximately 65 percent of these youngsters have skin blemishes severe enough to require medical treatment. About 50 percent of the entire population of the United States, 120 million people, will suffer from a cold or flu this year during the winter months alone. And another 60 percent is at this very moment stricken by some form of superficial fungal infection, such as athlete's foot or ringworm. The common ailments are very common indeed, and thousands of "cures" are promoted every year.

Unfortunately, with so many products marketed for the same ailments, it becomes increasingly difficult to know which ones work well, especially with the millions of advertising dollars that are invested annually to sway consumer attitudes. To make an intelligent choice, a knowledge of medicine and pharmacology is truly a prerequisite. It is my earnest hope that *Common Cures for Common Ailments* will deliver that knowledge. I have employed a question and answer format for the book, for I believe it is a technique that will help cut through the confusion about symptoms, both slight and serious, and their treatment with nonprescription, over-the-counter products.

Each chapter or section is devoted to a single ailment. The causes, symptoms, and courses of the ailment are described, and then the various generic drugs which can be used to cure the ailments are discussed. Finally, a list of all the available over-the-counter (OTC) products by brand names, including the ingredients of each, is presented so that consumers can make an intelligent choice for their own cure. In addition, I have noted with **boldface** which products are in my view the most appropriate. My evaluation is based on the recommendations of the Federal Drug Administration's panel on over-the-counter medications, manufacturers' claims, reviews in professional publications, and personal interviews.

Although I feel the book is very much needed by the average consumer, I also believe that it is just as sorely needed by medical practitioners. Most doctors have a good knowledge of pharmacology, especially with respect to the drugs they prescribe regularly. However, since they rarely come in contact with nonprescription products, many have only an inkling of their worth—in fact, few doctors even know what products are available to the public. Therefore, this book is also intended for doctors wishing to increase their knowledge of over-the-counter, nonprescription drugs.

A question that I frequently heard during the course of writing this book was: How safe are OTC products and do they really work? Although some over-the-counter drugs aren't worth a penny, the great majority are truly effective and, in many cases, contain the exact same ingredients found in more expensive prescription drugs. Over-the-counter medicines have been successfully tested on laboratory animals and selected human subjects long before being marketed to the general public and thus are certainly among the safest of all medications. Many have actually been prescription drugs that have proven to be safe and effective through years of use. All are approved by the Federal Drug Administration. Although there is some inherent risk in taking any drug, the ill effects of nonprescription drugs are extremely rare in view of the hundreds of millions of people who use these products daily.

Never before in the history of medicine in this country has the doctor been under such pressure from the medical consumer. Costs have skyrocketed as sophisticated equipment and techniques replace older and more simple means of diagnosing and treating illness. Malpractice has become a major problem facing both physicians and patients, for it often forces the doctor to practice defensive medicine and promotes higher professional fees and medical costs that are all ultimately passed on to the patients. Meanwhile, the public demands more information about their bodies and their illnesses, asking more questions about medical therapy and self-treatment. How can these questions be answered? How can these problems be solved?

As a physician, I have always recognized the need to inform the patient about his condition and the *various* means of treating it. Communication is the key to a good doctor-patient relationship and first-class health care. I am also aware of my own responsibilities as a physician and the personal responsibility we all bear for our own good health. With these thoughts in mind, *Common Cures for Common Ailments* was developed as a source book of medical information that allows every reader to assume a little more control over his or her health, thus leaving the physician free to deal with more serious medical problems. It is my hope that this book will not only direct medical consumers to proper self-therapy, but will also establish the good intentions of physicians everywhere and increase the overall quality of health in this country.

Here's how I would recommend the book to be used: For the information you want, go directly to the relevant chapter. It is not intended that you read the entire chapter; just read the answers to the questions that pertain to your situation. Pay close attention to the "Recommendations" and "Comments and Cautions" sections toward the end of each chapter, for therein lie the most direct route to the nonprescription drugs you need for your particular problem.

Review the drug list at the end of each chapter for specific brand names and ingredients. The products in **boldface** receive my personal endorsement. I believe they are the safest and most effective. They are preferred. Knowing that few pharmacies carry all the available choices, I have tried to endorse as many acceptable products as possible. While some lists have many preferred brands, other lists have only a few, maybe just one or two. Regardless, if you purchase any of the preferred products, you can be assured that you have selected the very best.

Albert Marchetti, M. D.
October 1978

Common Cures for Common Ailments

1. Aches and Pains

Does pain have a purpose?
Yes, pain does indeed have a purpose. It informs us that an insult or injury to body tissues is taking place and prompts us to remove the offending stimulus. When pain results from a burn, for example, we quickly withdraw from the heat in order to avoid continued damage. As our legs grow tired and sore after a long walk, pain will eventually force us to sit down and rest for a while. Thus, by indicating an immediate problem, pain often helps to prevent additional complications.

What are the different sensations of pain and why do they occur?
Pain is difficult to describe or even accurately remember, but several adjectives have been used to classify the different types. Aching pain most correctly expresses deep, prolonged, nagging pain such as the kind that accompanies bruises, strains, or sprains. Burning pain applies to the sensation we feel when our skin is damaged by heat. Pricking pain is realized when a sharp object, such as a pin or needle, is inserted into the body. These distinct pains are generated by various pain receptors throughout the body and are transmitted to the brain via different pain fibers, nerves. This is why they have individual qualities.

Why can one person tolerate more pain than another person?
In the past, it was thought that everyone had a different pain threshold; however, this is probably not true. Certainly,

1

social and familial conditionings play major roles in pain tolerance as exemplified by the stoic Greeks, who refused to acknowledge pain, and the proud American Indians, who also tried to ignore it. On the other hand, more emotional people might lose consciousness after experiencing a painful, although relatively insignificant, cut or burn. Thus, the response to pain is a conditioned reaction; we are each programmed to act the way we do.

Does the location of pain influence its sensation?
It absolutely does. Superficial pain, which is carried by large pain fibers originating on the body surface, is generally pricking in nature. It differs significantly from the deep or visceral pain that results from injury to the internal organs, because such inner pain travels by way of smaller pain fibers and usually has a dull aching quality. Pain in muscles and bones (musculoskeletal pain), which is also conducted by small nerve fibers, has a quality likened to visceral pain— deep, dull, and aching.

Pain originating in one place can frequently be felt in another area. Why does this happen?
When pain from one location is perceived in another location, it is called referred pain. Visceral and musculoskeletal pains are frequently felt on the surface of the body, instead of where they actually originate, and many times confuse the sufferer into thinking that the problem is superficial. Heart attacks, for example, refer pain to the neck, jaw, and left arm. Stomach pain may often be felt on the surface of the chest. Referred pain occurs because some pain fibers from muscles, bones, and organs crisscross in the brain with other pain fibers from the skin, and the mind cannot distinguish between the two.

How can pain be treated?
First, whatever is causing the pain should be removed, then appropriate therapy should be initiated. Most superficial aches and pains are effectively treated with over-the-counter pain relievers. Musculoskeletal and visceral pains are more

difficult to alleviate and, at times, require prescription drugs. Constant, severe, and unremitting pain may ultimately necessitate surgical disruption of the pain fibers that carry the tormenting sensations to the brain.

What over-the-counter drugs will effectively relieve aches and pains?

The OTC products that contain acetaminophen, phenacetin, aspirin, or salicylamide will all reduce minor aches and pains. The comparative effectiveness and possible side effects of these different ingredients are highly controversial.

Acetaminophen and phenacetin: These two closely related drugs are highly effective in relieving the minor aches and pains that are suffered daily. They are particularly useful in treating headaches, muscular pains that arise from excessive physical exertion or from colds and flus, and discomfort from injured, inflamed nerves. But, as antiinflammatory agents, they are inferior to aspirin and do not adequately eliminate the joint pains of arthritis and bursitis.

The most significant toxic effects of phenacetin include hemolytic anemia (a destruction of red blood cells that leads to abdominal pain and discomfort), fever, weakness, yellowing of the skin, and methemoglobin (a derangement in the oxygen-carrying protein found in red blood cells that results in difficult breathing, fatigue, nausea, vomiting, and a bluish purple discoloration of the lips, fingernails, and skin). Generally, the hemolytic anemias develop after prolonged phenacetin use. However, both hemolytic anemia and methemoglobin *can* occur after a single large ingestion of this drug. Negroes are more vulnerable to these side effects than Caucasians, and infants are more susceptible than grown-ups.

Acetaminophen rarely, if ever, causes the blood problems noted above, but it has been associated with abnormal blood clotting, which can appear both as excessive bruising or prolonged bleeding. In addition, severe liver disease, with its nausea, vomiting, abdominal pain, and skin yellowing (jaundice), has been reported in conjunction with massive acetaminophen ingestion. Other serious toxic reactions, kidney disease, low blood sugar, and heart muscle damage, have become a growing concern but, in view of the great number of people using this drug, these reactions are quite rare.

Aspirin: The pain-relieving qualities of aspirin are well recognized and have made this drug world renowned. Headaches, musclar soreness, and nerve tenderness all respond well to aspirin. Because aspirin reduces inflammation as well as alleviates pain, the bone and joint misery of rheumatoid arthritis and bursitis is greatly relieved when this medication is used. Unfortunately, it has several serious side effects.

Stomach irritation is common to aspirin users; so are such discomforts as heartburn and gastric upsets. Occasionally, tiny ulcers will form in the stomach lining, giving rise to bleeding and pain. When this happens, nausea and vomiting may occur, and the stools will become dark brown to brown-black.

Bleeding problems might also arise, since aspirin interrupts the normal clotting mechanism through an action on blood platelets and blood proteins.

Aspirin allergies exist too. They are recognized by the formation of hives, skin rashes, fever, and asthmalike reactions that quickly follow ingestion of the drug. Although these conditions are usually mild, a severe case can take the life of an unlucky victim. Asthma patients are particularly prone to aspirin allergies.

Poisonings from continued aspirin abuse are characterized by dizziness, personality change and confusion, headaches, and ringing in the ears. With a massive overdose, hyperventilation caused by rapid breathing will upset the normal acid-base balance of the body and can possibly produce convulsions and death.

Salicylamide: Although salicylamide is chemically similar to aspirin, it neither has the overall effectiveness nor the large number of toxic reactions. Unlike the other mild pain relievers, salicylamide exerts a mild depressant effect on the brain.

RECOMMENDED TREATMENT
Aspirin is the most widely used pain reliever on the market today, and rightfully so: it is an excellent drug with

many beneficial qualities. Generally, it is tolerated well by its users although the minor discomfort of stomach upset is fairly common. This can be avoided, however, by consuming buffered aspirin products or taking aspirin with milk.

Since no other nonprescription product can compare with aspirin in relieving the pain and discomfort of rheumatoid arthritis and bursitis, I highly recommend aspirin in these cases too. Headaches and the other minor aches and pains discussed are also easily treated with aspirin compounds.

Those people who cannot tolerate aspirin for any reason should use acetaminophen products. This includes anyone with aspirin allergies, asthma, bleeding tendencies, stomach ulcers, or chronic gastric irritation. Acetaminophen is also recommended for people on anticoagulant drugs, oral hypoglycemics (diabetic drugs), and medications for gout, where the concomitant use of aspirin might counter the intended effects of these other drugs.

COMMENTS AND CAUTIONS

I personally do not believe combination products provide greater relief than single-ingredient products, and I discourage their use because the potential hazard of developing an allergy to one of the ingredients overrides the possible, although unlikely, additive effects of such products.

Buffered aspirin products contain substances that decrease stomach acidity and, in so doing, promote rapid dissolution and absorption of the aspirin itself. This action prevents much of the gastric distress, because the aspirin does not remain in the stomach long enough to cause trouble.

Effervescent products that contain sodium bicarbonate also work well but, because of the high sodium concentration, they should not be used by people on salt-free diets.

Enteric-coated aspirin is designed to dissolve in the small intestine rather than in the stomach, thus avoiding possible gastric distress. Unfortunately, these products are erratically absorbed.

Time-released aspirins are acceptable, but one thing should be realized. Because these products dissolve slowly, they are not intended for the immediate relief of pain. Consequently, their use should be primarily limited to situations where continued aspirin therapy is required or for use at bedtime, when their time-releasing formula can provide adequate medication throughout the night.

Since most doctors and pharmacists believe that one brand of aspirin is as good as another, select the cheapest product after .comparing tablet strength, milligram for milligram.

MILD PAIN RELIEVERS
Boldface: Recommended

Actamin, tablet	acetaminophen
Act-On, tablet	sodium salicylate 194.3 mg salicylamide 129.6 mg potassium iodide sodium bicarbonate
Alka-Seltzer Effervescent Pain Reliever and Antacid	aspirin 325 mg sodium bicarbonate 1.904 g citric acid 1.0 g
Aluprin, tablet	aspirin 300 mg aluminum hydroxide gel magnesium hydroxide
Amphenol, tablet	acetaminophen 325 mg
Anacin, tablet	aspirin 400 mg caffeine 325 mg
Anacin, aspirin free tablet	acetaminophen 500 mg caffeine 32 mg
Anodynos, tablet	aspirin acetaminophen salicylamide caffeine

Apamide, tablet   acetaminophen 300 mg

Arthralgen, tablet   acetaminophen 250 mg
                                    salicylamide 250 mg

**Arthritis Pain   aspirin 486 mg
Formula, tablet**   aluminum hydroxide 20 mg
                                    magnesium hydroxide 60 mg

**Arthritis Strength   aspirin 486 mg
Bufferin, tablet**   magnesium carbonate 145.8 mg
                                    aluminum glycinate 72.9 mg

Arthropan, liquid   choline salicylate 870 mg/5 ml

A.S.A. Compound,   aspirin 227 mg
capsules   phenacetin 160 mg
                                    caffeine 32.5 mg

A.S.A. Enseals   aspirin 325 mg or 650 mg
                                    enteric coating

Ascriptin, tablet   aspirin 325 mg
                                    magnesium hydroxide 75 mg
                                    aluminum hydroxide gel 75 mg

**Ascriptin A/D,   aspirin 325 mg
tablet**   magnesium hydroxide 150 mg
                                    aluminum hydroxide gel 150 mg

Aspergum, gum   aspirin 228 mg

Azruman, tablet   salicylamide 260 mg
                                    potassium salicylate 228 mg

B-A, tablet   aspirin 325 mg
                                    aluminum hydroxide 100 mg
                                    magnesium hydroxide 20 mg

Bancap, capsule   acetaminophen 300 mg
                                    salicylamide 200 mg

**Bayer Aspirin,   Aspirin 325 mg
tablet**

Bayer Children's   aspirin 80 mg
aspirin, tablet

Bayer Non-Aspirin Pain Reliever, tablet   acetaminophen 325 mg

Bayer Timed-Release Aspirin, tablet   aspirin 650 mg

BC, tablet   aspirin 422 mg

BC, powder   aspirin 648 mg
salicylamide 194 mg

Bromo-Seltzer (per recommended dose)   acetaminophen 325 mg
phenacetin 130 mg
sodium bicarbonate/citric acid 2.8 g
caffeine 32.5 mg

Buffadyne, tablet   aspirin 230 mg
phenacetin 150 mg
caffeine 30 mg
aluminum hydroxide gel
magnesium hydroxide

Buffadyne 25, tablet   aspirin 230 mg
phenacetin 150
caffeine 30 mg
aluminum hydroxide gel
magnesium hydroxide
methapyrilene hydrochloride 25 mg

Buffaprin, tablet   aspirin
magnesium carbonate

Bufferin, tablet   aspirin 325 mg
magnesium carbonate 97.2 mg
aluminum glycinate 48.6 mg

Calurin, tablet   calcium carbaspirin

Cama, inlay-tab   aspirin 600 mg
magnesium hydroxide 150 mg
aluminum hydroxide gel 150 mg

Capital, tablet   acetaminophen 325 mg

Capron, capsule

aspirin 227 mg
acetaminophen 65 mg
phenacetin 162 mg
caffeine 32 mg

Comeback, tablet

acetaminophen 150 mg
salicylamide 150 mg
caffeine 100 mg

Cope, tablet

aspirin 421.2 mg
magnesium hydroxide 50 mg
caffeine 32 mg
aluminum hydroxide 25 mg
methapyrilene fumarate 12.5 mg

Cystex, tablet

salicylamide
methenamine
sodium salicylate
benzoic acid

Datril, tablet

acetaminophen 325 mg

**Datril Extra
Strength, tablet**

acetaminophen 500 mg

Dolcin, tablet

asprin 240.5 mg
calcium succinate 182 mg

Dolor, tablet

aspirin 230 mg
acetaminophen 230 mg
calcium carbonate 100 mg
skim milk powder 50 mg
caffeine 30 mg

Dularin, syrup

acetaminophen 120 mg/5 ml

Duradyne, tablet

aspirin 230 mg
acetaminophen 30 mg
phenacetin 150 mg
caffeine 15 mg

Duragesic, tablet

aspirin 325 mg
salicylic acid 162.5 mg

Ecotrin, tablet

aspirin 300 mg
enteric coating

Elixodyne, elixir	acetaminophen 120 mg alcohol 10%
Emagrin, tablet	aspirin salicylamide caffeine
Empirin Compound, tablet	aspirin 227 mg phenacetin 162 mg caffeine 32 mg
Excedrin, tablet	aspirin 194.4 mg acetaminophen 97 mg salicylamide 129.6 mg caffeine 64.8 mg
Excedrin P.M., tablet	aspirin 194.4 mg acetaminophen 162 mg salicylamide 129.6 mg methapyrilene fumarate 25 mg
Febrinol, tablet	acetaminophen 325 mg
Fendon, tablet	acetaminophen 325 mg
Fendon, elixir	acetaminophen 120 mg/5 ml alcohol 10%
Fizrin, powder,	aspirin 325mg sodium carbonate 400 mg sodium bicarbonate 1.825 g citric acid 1.449 g
Goody's Headache Powder	aspirin 455 mg phenacetin 325 mg caffeine 32.5 mg
Liquiprin, suspension	acetaminophen 699 mg/1.25 ml
Magan, tablet	magnesium salicylate 325 mg
Maranox, tablet	acetaminophen 60 mg salicylamide 150 mg phenacetin 100 mg caffeine 15 mg

Measurin, time-release, tablet   aspirin 650 mg

Medache, tablet   acetaminophen 150 mg
salicylamide 150 mg
phenyltoloxamine dihydrogen citrate
    44 mg
caffeine 32 mg

Nebs, tablet   acetaminophen 325 mg

Nebs, liquid   acetaminophen 120 mg/5 ml
alcohol 7%

Neocylate, tablet   potassium salicylate 280 mg
aminobenzoic acid 250 mg

Nilain, tablet   aspirin 325 mg
acetaminophen 162.5 mg
caffeine 32.5 mg

Nilprin 7½, tablet   acetaminophen 486 mg

Pabalate, tablet   sodium salicylate 300 mg
sodium aminobenzoate 300 mg

Pabalate SF, tablet   potassium salicylate 300 mg
potassium aminobenzoate 300 mg

Pabirin, tablet   aspirin 300 mg
aminobenzoic acid 300 mg
aluminum hydroxide gel 100 mg

PAC, capsule   aspirin 228 mg
phenacetin 163 mg
caffeine 32 mg

Panodyne, tablet   aspirin 260 mg
acetaminophen 64.8 mg
salicylamide 64.8 mg
caffeine 16.2 mg

Percogesic, tablet   acetaminophen 325 mg
phenyltoloxamine citrate 30 mg

Persistin, tablet   aspirin 160 mg
salicylsalicylic acid 485 mg

Pyradyne Comp., tablet	calicylamide 210 mg phenacetin 150 mg caffeine 30 mg pyrilamine maleate 15 mg
S-A-C, tablet	acetaminophen 150 mg salicylamide 230 mg caffeine 30 mg
Sal-Fayne, capsule	aspirin 228 mg phenacetin 166 mg caffeine 32 mg
Salicionyl, effervescent salt	sodium salicylate 650 mg/180 ml sodium carbonate 1.3 g/180 ml sodium and potassium citrates, tartrates, and malates
SK-APAP, tablets	acetaminophen 325 mg
SK-APAP, elixir	acetaminophen 120 mg/5 ml alcohol 8%
S.P.C., tablet	salicylamide 195 mg phenacetin 130 mg caffeine 16.25 mg
Stanback, tablet	aspirin 325 mg salicylamide 97 mg caffeine 16 mg
Stanback, powder	aspirin 648 mg salicylamide 194 mg caffeine 32 mg
Stanco Aspirin, tablet	aspirin 325 mg
St. Joseph Aspirin, tablet	aspirin 325 mg
St. Joseph Aspirin for Children, chewable tablet	aspirin 81 mg

St. Joseph Fever Reducer for Children, drops	acetaminophen 60 mg/0.6 ml alcohol 9.5%
St. Joseph Fever Reducer for Children, elixir	acetaminophen 120 mg/5 ml alcohol 7%
Strascogesic, tablet	acetaminophen 300 mg salicylamide 200 mg cellulose 102.7 mg alcohol 0.03 ml
Supac, tablet	aspirin 230 mg acetaminophen 160 mg caffeine 33 mg calcium gluconate 60 mg
Tempra, syrup	acetaminophen 120 mg/5 ml alcohol 10%
Tempra, tablet	acetaminophen 325 mg
Tempra, drops	acetaminophen 60 mg/0.6 ml alcohol 10%
Tenol, tablet	acetaminophen 325 mg
Trigesic Tablets	aspirin 230 mg acetaminophen 125 mg caffeine 30 mg
Tylaprin, elixir	acetaminophen 120 mg/5 ml alcohol 7%
Tylenol Extra Strength, tablet	acetaminophen 500 mg
Tylenol, tablet	acetaminophen 325 mg
Tylenol, drops	acetaminophen 60 mg/0.6 ml alcohol 7%
Tylenol, chewable tablet	acetaminophen 120 mg

Tylenol, liquid   acetaminophen 120 mg/5 ml
                             alcohol 7%

Uracel, tablet   sodium salicylate 325 mg

Valadol, tablet   acetaminophen 325 mg

Valadol, liquid   acetaminophen 120 mg/5 ml
                             alcohol 9%

Valorin, tablet   acetaminophen

Vanquish, caplet   aspirin 227 mg
                             acetaminophen 194 mg
                             magnesium hydroxide 50 mg
                             caffeine 33 mg
                             aluminum hydroxide gel 25 mg

2. Acne
(Blackheads and Pimples)

What is acne and why does it occur?
Acne is a skin problem that is characterized by pimples, pustules, and, in more severe cases, cysts that most frequently occur on the face, chest, and back of adolescent boys and girls. This condition arises when hormonal changes that come with puberty cause increased oil production in the thousands of sebaceous glands that are found throughout the skin. Sebaceous glands secrete a substance called sebum that protects and lubricates the surface of the skin. When these glands become clogged by oily plugs, acne results.

Who is affected by acne?
Although acne is not a serious problem, it is widespread. At least 75 percent of all adolescent boys and 50 percent of all adolescent girls will develop acne skin blemishes that are severe enough to treat. Unfortunately, acne cannot be cured, but with proper therapy it can be controlled.

What are some of the factors that contribute to acne problems?
There are quite a few contributory factors. Here are the most common ones.

Climate: Sunlight tends to prevent the development of oily skin plugs, but this beneficial effect is lost during the winter months when people remain indoors. Consequently, acne usually improves in the summer and worsens in the winter. Occasional flare-ups do occur in the summer, however, during periods of excessive heart and humidity, when sweating and skin irritation are frequent.

15

Cosmetics: Cosmetics can lead to acne lesions in two ways. First, by covering the skin, cosmetics seal off the small pores that allow oil to flow from the sebaceous glands. The stagnant oil will then thicken and form a plug which remains long after the cosmetic has been removed. Second, since some cosmetics are irritants, they can directly promote inflammation of the sebaceous glands and cause secondary eruptions.

Heredity: Physical qualities that are passed from parents to offspring will frequently be a factor. The number, size, shape, distribution, and activity of the sebaceous glands are all affected by heredity, and parents who have had acne problems are likely to have children with similar dilemmas.

Irritation: High school football players who use helmets and chin straps, laborers with heavy coveralls, and anyone else who must wear tight-fitting uniforms or clothing during the day tend to develop acne more readily than those who do not. Local irritation and the build-up of oil and grime are the causes.

Menstruation: During her menstrual period, a woman may notice that acne becomes worse. This occurs because progesterone, one of the female hormones that becomes active during the menses, increases sebaceous production and also narrows the sebaceous glands, thus facilitating obstruction and plugging.

Poor hygiene: If oil and dirt are allowed to build up on the skin, sebaceous glands will clog easily and pimples will result.

Does diet affect acne?

There is much discussion but little documented evidence that diet affects acne. Although foods like chocolate, cola, butter, and nuts have been implicated, clinical tests fail to show any direct correlation. Iodides and bromides, however, will produce acne if they are taken in excess, but the quantity of these substances found in normal diets is insufficient to cause any problems, There is a simple rule to follow: avoid any dietary food or product that seemingly has a bad effect on *your* skin.

How is acne best treated?
Treatment is directed at the underlying causes of this skin problem: excessive oil production and the clogged sebaceous glands.

Frequent washings constitute one of the most effective and least expensive means of controlling acne problems. In an attempt to remove excessive oil, all affected areas should be cleaned three times a day with warm water, soap, and a soft scrubbing aid such as a sponge or washcloth. Ordinary bath soap is quite adequate for daily use, but the soap should be completely rinsed from the skin with plenty of fresh water. Soapy residues that remain on the skin can cause additional irritation. Medicated soaps are expensive and probably no more effective than ordinary soap because, with rinsing, the active ingredients are removed from the skin and therefore cannot provide additional benefit.

Since sunlight prevents plugging and promotes sebaceous drainage, sun exposure should be sought whenever possible. Sun lamps can also be helpful, but must be used cautiously; serious burns can debilitate overzealous users.

Topical lotions and creams that prevent plugging of the sebaceous glands are extremely useful and have been proven effective. They promote mild skin peeling and rapid cell-growth rates, two actions that keep oil ducts open by removing old sticky cells and allowing young healthy cells to regrow in their place. By combining frequent washings, sun exposure, and topical antiacne lotions and creams, annoying skin blemishes can be greatly reduced and the development of new blemishes can be arrested.

What medications are available without a prescription?
There are four major kinds of OTC medications that are used for treating acne.

Benzoyl peroxide: Benzoyl peroxide is an irritating agent that cleans out sebaceous glands and stimulates new cell growth. It is used by many leading dermatologists on their acne patients.

Resorcinol and salicylic acid: These two antiacne medications are frequently used in combination and, basically, have the same effect as benzoyl peroxide. However, they are not as strong.

Sulfur: Sulfur is found in numerous OTC products and helps to reduce acne blemishes. Unfortunately, it sometimes causes new pimple formation; therefore, its use is currently being questioned.

Topical antibacterial compounds: Iodine, phenol, methylbenzethonium chloride, hydroxyquinoline, and chloroxylenol are the antibacterial agents found in acne products. They will diminish the bacteria present on the skin, but their effect is short lived. Furthermore, since bacteria play an insignificant role in the development of ordinary acne, the indications for their use are somewhat limited.

RECOMMENDED TREATMENT

Adequate skin hygiene is of the utmost importance, and frequent washings are a must. In mild cases, skin cleansing may be all that is needed to keep acne in check. However, when mild to moderate acne is a problem, resorcinol and salicylic acid will prove helpful. These agents should be used in 2 percent creams or lotions combined in an alcohol base. The alcohol not only promotes quick drying, but it also reduces the swelling that frequently closes oil ducts.

Occasionally, medication that is stronger than salicylic acid and resorcinol is necessary, in which case benzoyl peroxide should be used. Products with a 5 percent concentration should be tried initially, and the stronger 10 percent products should be reserved for more difficult cases and hardier skin. With normal use, this medication will produce a slight burning sensation, although excessive stinging may occur with a single application. Whenever burning is extreme, the medication should be removed by washing, and treatment should be resumed the following day. If redness, dryness, or peeling becomes overwhelming, the use of benzoyl peroxide should be briefly discontinued.

COMMENTS AND CAUTIONS

In the past, antibiotics such as tetracycline and erythromycin have been randomly used to treat acne, but presently they are reserved only for severe inflammatory acne conditions. Inflammatory acne is recognized by large, firm pustules and nodules that occur beneath the skin and are associated with tenderness, redness, and scar formation. Since bacteria are thought to play a prominent role in the development of inflammatory acne, antibiotics have been used in the treatment of this severe condition. Eliminating the causative bacteria is best accomplished by taking oral erythromycin or tetracycline, antibiotics that are available by prescription only. The antibacterial action of these drugs far surpasses the effect of over-the-counter antibiotic lotions, but their general use is not recommended. Instead, most physicians advise their patients to follow a conscientious program of daily washings combined with the application of salicylic acid, resorcinol, or benzoyl peroxide.

If your complexion problem is confined to your face, chest, or back and consists of pimples and blackheads only, self-medication is advisable. However, if you notice red, swollen nodules and cysts, or skin sores that appear on other parts of your body, see your doctor.

Also, certain ingredients found in acne preparations (resorcinol and benzoyl peroxide) may cause pale areas to develop on dark skin. Consider this before using these products.

ANTIACNE MEDICATIONS
Boldface: Recommended

Acnaveen, cream	salicylic acid 2% sulfur 2% soapless detergents
Acne Aid, cream	resorcinol 1.25% sulfur 2.5% chloroxylenol 0.375%

Acne Aid, lotion

sulfur 10%
alcohol 10%

Acne-Aid Detergent
Soap

surface active cleanser
hydrocarbon hydrotropes 6.3%

Acne Cream

sulfur
resorcinol
zinc oxide
para-chloro-meta-zylenol
alcohol 9.25%

Acnederm, lotion

sulfur 5%
zinc oxide 10%
zinc sulfate 1%

Acne-Dome Creme
and Lotion

resorcinol monoacetate
sulfur

Acne-Dome
Medicated Cleanser

salicylic acid
sulfur

Acnesarb, solution

salicylic acid 3%
methylbenzethonium chloride 0.08%
isopropyl alcohol 63%
boric acid 2%

Acnomel, cream

resorcinol 2%
sulfur 8%
alcohol 11%
grease-free vehicle

Acnomel, cake

resorcinol 1%
sulfur 4%

Acnomel, cleanser

resorcinol 1%
sulfur 4%

Acnotex, lotion

salicylic acid 2.25%
sulfur 8%
methylbenzethonium chloride 0.08%
propylene glycol
powder base
acetone
isopropyl alcohol 22%
perfume

Acnycin, cream	resorcinol 2% sulfur 5% zinc oxide
Alphcene Cleanser	resorcinol sulfur
Bare Face, acne **skin medicine,** **foam**	salicylic acid resorcinol alcohol benzalkonium chloride
Benoxyl, lotion	benzoyl peroxide 5%–10%
Bensulfoid, lotion	resorcinol 2% sulfur 2% alcohol 12% zinc oxide 6% thymol 0.5% hexachlorophene 0.1% perfume
Betadine, skin cleanser	povidone-iodine 7.5% detergents
Brade-A-Foam	pumice scrub
Brasivol, cleanser	aluminum oxide neutral soap detergents (fine, medium, rough)
Cenac, lotion	resorcinol 2% sulfur 8% isopropyl alcohol 30%
Clearasil, medicated cleanser	salicylic acid 0.25% alcohol 43% allantoin 0.1%
Clearasil, cream	resorcinol 2% sulfur 8% bentonite 11% alcohol 10%
Clearasil, stick	resorcinol 1% bentonite 4%

Clearasil Antibacterial Lotion

benzoyl peroxide 5%

Clearasil Vanishing Formula, cream

resorcinol 2%
sulfur 3%
bentonite 10%
alcohol 10%

Contrablem, gel

resorcinol 2%
sulfur 5%
alcohol 9.5%

Cuticura, ointment

sulfur
8-hydroxyquinoline
petrolatum
mineral oil
mineral wax
isopropyl palmitate
synthetic beeswax
phenol
pine oil
rose geranium oil

Cuticura Acne Cream

benzoyl peroxide 5%
alcohol 1%

Cuticura Medicated Liquid

salicylic acid
resorcinol
8-hydroxyquinoline sulfate
phenol
alcohol 28%
boric acid
chlorobutanol
camphor

Dry & Clear, lotion

benzoyl peroxide 5%

Epi-Clear, lotion for acne

benzoyl peroxide 5%–10%

Epi-Clear, lotion

sulfur 10%
alcohol 10%

Epi-Clear, scrub cleanser

aluminum oxide (fine 38%, medium 52%, coarse 65%)

Epi-Clear, soap for oily skin	sulfated surface active cleanser 6.3% hydrocarbon hydrotropes
Exzit Cleanser	salicylic acid sulfur
Exzit Creme/Lotion	resorcinol sulfur
Finac, lotion	sulfur 2% methylbenzethonium chloride 0.08% powder base isopropyl alcohol 8% perfume
Fomac, cream cleanser	salicylic acid 2% sulfur 2% soapless detergents
Fomac-HF, cleanser	chloroxylenol 2%
Fostex Acne Gel	benzoyl peroxide 5%
Fostex Medicated Cleanser	benzoyl peroxide 5% sulfur 2% wetting agents
Ionax Foam, aerosol foam	benzalkonium chloride 0.2% polyoxyethylene ethers surface active cleanser
Ionax Scrub, paste	benzalkonium chloride 0.2% polyethylene granules polyoxyethylene ethers alcohol 10%
Klaron, lotion	salicylic acid 2% sulfur 5% alcohol 13.1%
Komed, lotion	salicylic acid 2% resorcinol 2% isopropyl alcohol 22% sodium thiosulfate 8% menthol camphor colloidal alumina

Komex, cleanser | sodium tetrahydrate decahydrate granules

Liquimat, lotion | sulfur 5%
alcohol 22%
tinted bases

Listerex Herbal Lotion, cleanser | salicylic acid 2%
polyethylene granules
surface active cleansers

Listerex Regular Lotion, cleanser | thymol 0.16%
polyethylene granules
surface active cleansers
menthol
eucalyptol

Loroxide, lotion | chlorhydroxyquinoline 0.25%
benzoyl peroxide 5%

Lotio Alsulfa, lotion | sulfur 5%
clays 0.05%

Lotioblanc, lotion | zinc sulfate
sulfurated potash

Medicated Face Conditioner "MFC," lotion | salicylic acid 1%
alcohol 55%

Microsyn, lotion | salicylic acid 2%
resorcinol 2%
sodium thisosulfate 8%
colloidal alumina
menthol
camphor

Multiscrub, cream | salicylic acid 1.5%
sulfur 2%
soapless detergents
polyethylene resin granules 26%

Neutrogene Acne Drying Gel | isopropyl alcohol 47%
gel base

Neutrogena Acne Soap	triethanolamine glycerin fatty acids acetulan tea lauryl sulfate
Oxy Scrub	dissolving abradant particles sodium tetraborate decahydrate
Oxy-5, lotion	benzoyl peroxide 5%
Pernox	salicylic acid 1.5% sulfur 2% oil base
Persadox, lotion	benzoyl pcroxide 5%
Persadox HP, cream	benzoyl peroxide 10%
phisoAc, cream	resorcinol 1.5% sulfur 6% alcohol 10%
pHisoDan	sulfur 5% sodium salicylate 0.5% oil base
pHisoDerm, cleanser	entsufon sodium petrolatum lanolin cholesterols
piSec, cream	sulfur 3.14% benzalkonium chloride 0.2% polyoxyethylene ethers
Postacne, lotion	sulfur 2% alcohol 29%
Propathymol P.H., lotion	benzoic acid boric acid thymol eucalyptol alcohol 28%

Quinalor Compound, ointment	halquinols 0.5% benzoyl peroxide 10% menthol methyl salicylate polyethylene glycol mineral oil
Resulin, lotion	resorcinol 4% sulfur 8% alcohol 32%
Rezamid, lotion	resorcinol 2% sulfur 5% chloroxylenol 0.5% alcohol 28.5%
Sastid Plain, cleanser	salicylic acid 1.6% sulfur 1.6% surface active cleanser aluminum oxide
Seale's, lotion	resorcinol 3.2% sulfur 6.5% sodium borate zinc oxide acetone bentonite
Seba-Nil, solution	alcohol 49.7% acetone polysorbate 80
Seba-Nil Cleansing Mask	polyethylene granules
Spectro-Jel, gel	cetylpyridinium chloride 0.1% isopropyl alcohol 15% methylcellulose 1.5% glycol-polysiloxane 1%
Stri-Dex Medicated Pads	salicylic acid 0.5% sulfonated alkylbenzenes citric acid alcohol

Sulforcin, lotion	resorcinol 2% sulfur 5% alcohol 11.65%
Sulfur, soap	sulfur 10%
Teenac, gel	sulfur 1.5% mercuric sulfide 0.5% urea
Ten-O-Six Acne Blemish Cream	resorcinol sulfur isopropyl alcohol 38.5% allantoin panthenol galacturonic acid
Thera-Blem, cream	resorcinol 1.5% sulfur 2% phenol 0.5% menthol 0.5% camphor 0.5% oil base
Therac, lotion	salicylic acid 2.35% sulfur 4% bentonite perfume
Therapads	salicylic acid 1.5% alcohol 50%
Therapads Plus	salicylic acid 1.5% alcohol 70% sodium alkyl aryl polyether sulfonate 0.1%
Thylox Medicated Soap	sulfur 8.8%
Topex, lotion	benzoyl peroxide 10%
Transact, lotion	sulfur 2% laureth-4 6%

Tyrosum Packets,   alcohol
cleanser   acetone
                          polysorbate

Vanoxide, lotion   chlorhydroxyquinoline 0.25%
                          benzoyl peroxide 5%

Xerac, gel   sulfur 4%
                          isopropyl alcohol 44%

3. Allergies
(Allergic Rhinitis, Hayfever, and Hives)

What is allergic rhinitis?
Allergic rhinitis is an inflammatory reaction that occurs in the nose and sinuses. It is characterized by sneezing and itching, nasal congestion and swelling, plus thin, watery mucus which runs from the nose.

Are there different types of allergic rhinitis?
Yes, there are. When the condition is caused by airborne pollen from trees, grass, ragweed, and other similar pollenating plants, it is called seasonal allergic rhinitis, or hayfever, and occurs primarily in the spring and summer. If the reaction is noted throughout the year and is related to allergens other than pollen, it is called nonseasonal or perennial (yearly) allergic rhinitis.

What are the different seasons and causes for hayfever?
Spring hayfever, occurring in April and May, is usually due to tree pollen. Summer hayfever, which occurs in June and July, probably results from exposure to pollens from grass. And, finally, late-summer allergic rhinitis is a reaction to weed pollen.

What is pollen?
Some plants, like most animals, have male and female sexes and multiply by sexual reproduction. Spores, which are grown on the male plant, are carried by insects or by the

wind to waiting female plants which are then impregnated. Pollen is the name given to masses of male spores.

How does pollen, dust, and other allergens cause allergic rhinitis?
The air which we breathe contains many impurities. One of the functions of the nose is to filter out these impurities and protect the lungs. As pollen, dust, and other inhaled allergens pass through the nose, they are trapped in the nasal mucus and are thus removed from the air. Unfortunately, some people react adversely to the presence of these substances and set a natural defense mechanism into operation. This mechanism, which involves the production of antibodies against the pollen or dust, give rise to the symptoms of allergic rhinitis.

Who is affected?
Approximately 10 percent of the population is affected by hayfever although not all of these people need treatment.

What are the symptoms of hayfever?
Nasal swelling and congestion are the commonest symptoms. They are caused by widening of the numerous small blood vessels in the nose and the loss of fluid from these blood vessels into the nasal lining, which forces the lining to swell. Itching within the nose is also common and gives rise to sudden and massive sneeze attacks. The flow of thin, watery mucus is excessive.

Can the eyes be affected?
Yes, pollen can be carried into the eyes, just as it is breathed through the nose, and, once inside the eyelids, produces the same swelling, redness, itching, and congestion that occurs in the nose.

What is the fate of the hayfever sufferer?
Most people who suffer from allergic rhinitis or hayfever notice that the illness gets progressively worse for a few years, but eventually it moves into a stable pattern which

occurs seasonally or yearly on a permanent basis. Some hayfever sufferers, possibly as many as 30 percent, will go on to experience other diseases such as allergic asthma. Still others may develop allergic complications, which include inflammation and irritation of the sinuses or ears, and nasal polyps, small soft grapelike swellings that are caused by the excessive collection of fluid in the lining of the nose and sinuses.

Are nasal polyps dangerous?
While nasal polyps are not dangerous, a doctor should be notified when they are noticed.

What is the treatment for allergic rhinitis?
There are three major components of effective allergy therapy. First, whenever possible, an attempt must be made to avoid the specific allergen: pollen, dust, animal hair, and so forth. Avoid trips to the country during allergy season, get rid of the pets, and thoroughly dust and air the house (or, better yet, have someone else do it). Use your own good judgment and common sense here. Second, lessen the severity of symptoms with effective allergy medication. Third, in extreme cases, desensitization therapy from a doctor may be indicated.

Who should be desensitized?
Since most people who suffer from allergic rhinitis experience only minor discomfort and can obtain relief with allergy medication, desensitization is usually not needed. However, for those people who have prolonged severe symptoms, lasting throughout the entire allergy season, and who cannot be relieved by allergy products, a doctor's evaluation and possibly desensitization should be sought.

What medication can be taken to relieve allergy symptoms?
Antihistamines are very effective drugs for symptomatic relief of allergic rhinitis, especially the seasonal variety, such as hayfever.

How do they work?

As previously mentioned, people who suffer from allergic rhinitis respond to the presence of pollen or other allergens by setting one of the body's natural defense mechanisms into operation. This mechanism involves the interaction between the allergen and the antibodies produced by the body. As a result of that interaction, a substance called histamine is released from cells within the body and causes blood vessels to increase in size, leak fluid, and produce edema. Antihistamines block the action of histamines and prevent its harmful effects.

Can antihistamines prevent allergy symptoms

Partially. Antihistamines block the action of histamines by covering the "sites" where histamine works, in blood vessels, glands, and muscles. For example, histamine often makes blood vessels increase in size. Antihistamines will attach themselves to the same receptor sites and prevent histamine from working there, in this case reducing the size of the blood vessel.

Antihistamines can be taken *before* exposure to pollen or dust in order to block histamine receptor-sites and thus prevent allergic symptoms. Although histamine is still released as the individual is exposed to the allergen, it cannot exert its full effect because the receptor sites are occupied by antihistamine drugs.

What antihistamines are available in over-the-counter medications?

The following list indicates the antihistamines which are available over-the-counter. Each is effective if used in the proper dose. Unfortunately, they are usually found in combination products that contain decongestants, stimulants, and mild pain relievers.

brompheniramine
chlorpheniramine
diphenhydramine

doxylamine
methapyrilene
phenindamine
pheniramine
pyrilamine
thonzylamine

Which is the best antihistamine?

The antihistamines listed above are equally effective in blocking the action of histamine, but they have variable side effects, the most significant of which is drowsiness. Brompheniramine, chlorpheniramine, and pheniramine produce the least drowsiness while diphenhydramine and doxylamine produce the most. Therefore, for daytime use I recommend the first three. In the evening, when a sedative effect may be desired, diphenhydramine or doxylamine can be taken.

RECOMMENDED TREATMENT

An allergy-combating product that contains an antihistamine in adequate dosage and a minimum amount of other products is recommended. The decongestants found in the numerous combination-products will reduce nasal congestion, but, when it is particularly bothersome, relief can be obtained by nasal-decongestant sprays or drops. A detailed discussion about decongestants can be found in Chapter 7, "Colds and Flus" (pages 59-62, 64-65, 66).

COMMENTS AND CAUTIONS

There are always precautions associated with drug use. Whenever possible, antihistamines should not be taken with alcohol, sedatives, strong pain-killers, or tranquilizers. *Nor should they be used by pregnant or nursing women.*

Antihistamines may become ineffective with continued use. If you find this to be true, change drugs. Frequently, the new drug will produce much better results and if it, too, loses its effectiveness with time, the first drug or another new antihistamine, may be tried again.

A doctor should be consulted if symptoms are debilitating or if complications such as asthma or inflammatory polyps occur.

DECONGESTANT MEDICATIONS

For a listing of decongestants, please turn to Chapter 7, "Colds and Flus" (pages 84-98).

4. Animal Bites

Are animal bites serious?
For the most part, animal bites pose no great risk to general health. Although the wounds require treatment, serious complications are rare.

What are the possible consequences of animal bites?
The greatest fear is the possibility of rabies, a viral disease that attacks the brain. While the fear of the disease may be great, the disease itself is rarely contracted.

Rabies is predominantly carried by wild animals, such as foxes, skunks, squirrels, and wolves, and infrequently by domestic animals, such as dogs and cats. Immunizations protect most pets, but occasionally these too become infected.

If you are bitten, there are several things to be observed.
(1) Did the animal act strangely and attack without provocation?
(2) Was the animal foaming at the mouth?
(3) Was the animal wild?

If the answer to any of these questions is yes, consider the possibility of rabies. If the answers are no, you have little to worry about. But remember, even domestic animals should be observed for two weeks; so, if the owner refuses to observe the animal, have it quarantined for that purpose.

Other possible consequences of animal bites include severe lacerations with scarring and infection.

RECOMMENDED TREATMENT
If rabies is not suspected, animal bites should be treated like any other lacerations or cuts. Large wounds that

require sutured closure obviously must be directed to a doctor or emergency service. Otherwise, smaller wounds can be self-treated.

Wash these wounds immediately with soap and water, then sterilize them with an antiseptic and dress them with an antibiotic cream or ointment. Daily hot-water soaks, three times a day for thirty minutes, will help to prevent infection of larger, deeper wounds. If infection does occur, see your doctor.

COMMENTS AND CAUTIONS
If rabies is suspected, call your doctor immediately. Rabies vaccine and antirabies serum may be necessary.

ANTIBIOTIC CREAMS AND OINTMENTS
For a listing of these medications, please turn to Chapter 11, "Cuts, Scrapes, and Scratches" (pages 143-44).

5. Asthma

What is asthma?
Asthma is an illness characterized by the narrowing of the air passages (trachea and bronchi) that lead to the lungs and the air tubes present within the lungs themselves (bronchioles).

Who is affected by asthma?
Approximately 2 to 3 percent of the population of the United States has asthma symptoms, or approximately six million people. One-half of these people are children under ten years of age.

What causes asthma?
There are numerous factors which are associated with asthma attacks, and these include physical and chemical irritants, psychological factors, nervousness, physical exertion, and infection. Here is a general review of each factor.

Physical and Chemical Irritants: This list is lengthy, so I will mention only a select number of irritants. I am sure different people react to different irritants in their own way, and substances not mentioned here or in expanded reports can cause asthmatic reactions in certain susceptible individuals. Specific irritants commonly associated with asthma include household dust; industrial products and pollutants, such as sulfur dioxide and aluminum flux; toluene isocyonate; pollens; and animal hair and dander.

Psychological and Nervous Factors: Normally, the trachea and bronchi narrow in response to stress and tension.

People with asthma have very sensitive tracheas and bronchi; they have an exaggerated response and become excessively narrow if they are stimulated. Consequently, if an asthmatic is placed in a stressful situation, heightened emotions might lead to excessive narrowing of these vital air passages.

Physical Exertion: For unknown reasons, asthmatic attacks can occur following excessive physical activity, especially in children and young adults. Interestingly, bronchoconstriction (a narrowing of the air passages) following exercise may be the first sign of asthma in many people who go on to experience more generalized asthmatic attacks.

Infections: Infections of the respiratory tract, common colds, bronchitis, laryngitis, and pneumonia, are frequently associated with asthma attacks. These attacks could simply be the result of an excessive reaction to the infection, or they may actually represent an allergic response to chemical factors of the virus or toxins released during the infection.

Are there different types of asthma?
Possibly. People who suffer from asthma fall into two broad categories. The first category includes children and young adults who have allergic diseases, such as hayfever, positive allergy skin tests, increased antibodies in the blood, and family members who have similar allergic problems. The second category consists of middle-aged people who have no hayfever, no positive skin tests, no increased antibodies, and no family members with allergies or asthma. This second group, however, is sensitive to aspirin. The first group is referred to as allergic asthmatics or extrinsic asthmatics. The second group is called nonallergic asthmatics or intrinsic asthmatics. Although not everyone falls perfectly into one of these two categories, generally the classification is valid.

Can asthma be considered a true allergy?
Yes and no. An allergy is an illness which occurs after exposure to a specific substance to which a person is sensi-

tive. Allergies are associated with an increase in antibodies and specific symptoms caused by the release of histamine, a naturally occurring substance in the body. People with allergic or extrinsic asthma seem to have real allergic reactions that appear as asthma. People who fall into the nonallergic- or intrinsic-asthma category evidently do not have this allergic component to their asthma.

What are the signs and symptoms of asthma?
Asthma usually appears quickly, beginning with a feeling of tightness in the chest, coughing, and wheezing. The difficulty in breathing that follows occurs because the passages in the lungs become very narrow, especially when air is being exhaled. Consequently, the lungs fill with air but cannot easily be deflated.

What is wheezing?
Wheezing is the whistling sound that comes from the narrow air passages in the lung as air is forced through them.

Can asthma symptoms be confused with other medical problems?
Yes. Chronic bronchitis, emphysema, lung infections, lung cancer, and even common respiratory-tract illnesses, such as colds and flus can be confused with asthma.

How can asthma be distinguished from these other ailments.?
Usually, these other ailments have prolonged, continuous symptoms rather than the interrupted, episodic reactions which characterize asthma.

Should anyone with asthma symptoms treat themselves?
No! Only people who have been diagnosed as asthmatics should treat themselves for that illness.

**Should asthmatics be under the supervision
of a doctor?**
Absolutely! Asthma is a serious illness and can cause death
to people who ignore its dangers. A doctor's supervision is
essential in directing the asthmatic and controlling his
disease.

Who should use over-the-counter asthma products?
People who have mild to moderate asthma and are under a
doctor's supervision can safely use OTC asthma products for
quick relief of symptoms. However, if those symptoms become worse and prolonged, the doctor should be consulted
immediately. Also, if OTC products do not provide satisfac-
tory results, they should not be used again. Once more a call
to the doctor is advised.

Are there different products available?
Yes, products which can be taken by mouth or inhaled are
available.

**What are the antiasthmatic drugs found in over-the-
counter oral preparations?**
There are two, ephedrine and theophylline.
   Ephedrine: Ephedrine counteracts the narrowing of the
air passages in the lungs by causing the small muscles that
surround the bronchi and bronchioles to relax and expand.
This is known as bronchodilation.
   Ephedrine does have several characteristic side effects. It
may increase blood pressure, cause the heart to beat faster
and stronger, produce nervousness or anxiety, and possibly
promote insomnia. Difficulty in passing urine may be noted
in older men with prostrate enlargement. Also, a rise in
blood sugar may occur after taking this drug, so diabetics
should monitor urine sugar.
   Since ephedrine requires up to one hour to work, it is best
used to prevent asthma attacks that can be anticipated.
Ephedrine acts too slowly to have any effect on acute
asthma symptoms.

Theophylline: This drug is a very powerful bronchodilator that causes the smooth muscles that surround the trachea, bronchi, and bronchioles to relax and widen, as ephedrine does. And like ephedrine, it also has several characteristic side effects. It will stimulate skeletal muscle and heart muscle, enlarge the blood vessels of the heart, and increase kidney activity.

Also, significant side effects, which are usually associated with excessive use of this drug, occur. These include loss of appetite, nausea, vomiting, and—in more severe cases—convulsions, coma, and shock. The more severe reactions have primarily been noted in children who have received excessively large doses.

Theophylline can be purchased over the counter in several different preparations, which usually contain other drugs as well. For example, many OTC products contain ephedrine and phenobarbital in addition to theophylline. (Phenobarbital is a depressant drug which is intended to counteract the stimulation caused by ephedrine.)

What is the medication found in inhalant preparations?
Epinephrine is found in the inhalant OTC products and is very effective in causing bronchodilation within a few minutes after administration. Unfortunately, it is not a long-acting drug and must be used repeatedly.

Are there unwanted side effects noted with epinephrine use?
Yes, there are. Nervousness, jitters, sleeplessness, dry mouth and throat, stomach upsets, anxiety, and heart palpitations have been reported. The least significant of these, dry mouth and throat, can be prevented by rinsing the mouth with water or mouthwash after the inhaler is used. The other side effects are usually related to the amount of medication consumed and vary from person to person.

How should inhalants be used?
Before using inhalants, or any other form of medication, the instructions provided with the product should be read carefully and followed precisely. Inhalants are generally used in the following manner. (1) All air is forced from the lungs. (2) The inhaler is held upside down and placed in the mouth with the teeth and lips holding and sealing the mouthpiece. (3) The head is slightly tilted backward. (4) The inhaler is activated after a deep breath has started, and is used continuously through a long smooth inhalation. (5) At the end of the inhalation, the inhaler is removed from the mouth, and the air is held within the lungs as long as it is comfortable to do so. It is then slowly expelled.

How should oral products be used?
These products should not be taken for acute attacks because they take too long to work. However, they can be used to counteract prolonged symptoms. They should be taken in recommended dosages at the appropriate time intervals, with the final dose taken just before bedtime, since asthma attacks are common at night.

RECOMMENDED TREATMENT
For acute attacks, I recommend epinephrine inhalants. For mild-to-moderate, continuous asthma symptoms, I recommend ephedrine and, for more severe continued asthmatic attacks, I recommend theophylline.

COMMENTS AND CAUTIONS
The continued use of epinephrine can lead to a drug tolerance that, in turn, leads to an increase in the amount of drug needed to produce the bronchodilation that relieves asthma attacks. By increasing the amount of epinephrine, side effects become more frequent. And, ultimately, the

drug may completely fail to provide adequate relief. These points are emphasized because, when noted, they should prompt the asthmatic to seek professional medical assistance immediately.

People who suffer from heart disease, high blood pressure, or thyroid disease should not use epinephrine unless they are advised to do so by their doctor. People who have asthma-like symptoms but have not been diagnosed as asthmatics should not use this drug either.

The best way to control asthma is to avoid any allergens, irritants, or stressful situations associated with your attacks. Undertaking these measures may provide complete relief and prevent the appearance of future symptoms. Desensitization might be an alternative for those who suffer from allergic asthma, but a doctor's evaluation is essential in this regard.

For relief from continuous and prolonged mild attacks, ephedrine or theophylline should be taken by mouth or used in suppository form.

Adequate hydration is another very important component of effective asthma therapy. At least one quart of water should be drunk daily by people who are experiencing asthma symptoms.

ASTHMA MEDICATIONS
Boldface: Recommended

Amodrine, tablet

    ephedrine 25 mg
    aminophylline 100 mg
    phenobarbital 8 mg

Asma-Lief, tablet

    ephedrine 24 mg
    theophylline 130 mg
    phenobarbital 8 mg

Bronitin, tablet

    ephedrine 24 mg
    theophylline 130 mg
    guaifenesin 100 mg
    methapyrilene 16 mg

Bronkaid, tablet

ephedrine 24 mg
theophylline 100 mg
guaifenesin 100 mg
magnesium trisilicate 74.52 mg

Bronkotabs, tablet

ephedrine 24 mg
theophylline 100 mg
guaifenesin 100 mg
phenobarbital 8 mg

Phedral, tablet

ephedrine 24.3 mg
theophylline 129.6 mg
phenobarbital 8.1 mg

Primatene M, tablet

ephedrine 24 mg
theophylline 130 mg
methapyrilene 16 mg

**Primatene P,
tablet**

ephedrine 24 mg
theophylline 130 mg
phenobarbital 8 mg

Tedral, tablet

ephedrine 24 mg
theophylline 130 mg
phenobarbital 8 mg

Tedral, elixir

ephedrine 6 mg/5 ml
theophylline 32.5 mg/5 ml
phenobarbital 2 mg/5 ml

Tedral, suspension

ephedrine 12 mg/5 ml
theophylline 65 mg/5 ml
phenobarbital 4 mg/5 ml

Thalfed, tablet

ephedrine 25 mg
theophylline 120 mg
phenobarbital 8 mg

Verequad, tablet

ephedrine 24 mg
theophylline 130 mg
guaifenesin 100 mg
phenobarbital 8 mg

Verequad, suspension	ephedrine 12 mg/5 ml theophylline 65 mg/5 ml guaifenesin 50 mg/5 ml phenobarbital 4 mg/5 ml

INHALERS

Asthma Haler	epinephrine 7 mg/ml
Asthma Nefrin	epinephrine 2.25% chlorobutanol 0.5%
Breatheasy	epinephrine 2.2% benzyl alcohol 1% isotonic salts 0.5%
Bronkaid mist	epinephrine 0.5% ascorbic acid 0.07% alcohol 34% hydrochloric and nitric acid buffers
Primatene Mist	epinephrine 0.2 mg/5 ml
Vaponefrin Solution	epinephrine 2.25% chlorobutanol 0.5%

6. Burns

How common are burns?

Burns account for about 8,000 deaths in the United States each year, with many of the fatalities occurring among young children. Millions of other Americans receive burns of lesser severity and, although many of these people require hospitalization or professional medical attention, the majority can adequately treat themselves.

Exactly what happens when you are burned?

The simplest way to answer that question is to say your body tissues become cooked when burned in a minor way and actually charred when severely burned. Excessive heat causes the proteins present within body tissue to jell or curdle, which in turn produces the death and destruction of the tissue. Blood vessels, which are needed to carry life-sustaining nutrients and oxygen to all living body parts, may be destroyed in a burn, and this can result in the death of the skin or tissue supplied by those blood vessels. Lesser damage to blood vessels will cause them to leak fluid and, in this way, blisters are formed.

How are burns classified?

Burns are classified in three major subdivisions.

First-degree, or superficial burns: Superficial burns involve only the upper layer of the skin, the epidermis, and leave skin accessories such as hair follicles, sweat glands, and oil glands untouched.

Second-degree, or partial-thickness, burns: Partial-thickness burns involve not only the epidermis, but the skin accessories as well. Although the hair follicles and sweat glands are not destroyed in second-degree burns, they may be severely damaged and usually require weeks for regrowth. These burns, under normal circumstances, will heal completely.

Third-degree, or full-thickness, burns: Full-thickness burns extend deeply into the skin and beyond. The epidermis and the accessory skin structures are completely destroyed, leaving severe, open, draining wounds. The underlying subcutaneous fat and blood vessels are also destroyed or badly injured, causing prolonged and often incomplete wound healing.

In superficial and partial-thickness burns, the skin will regrow from the cells lining the hair follicles and accessory glands; but in full-thickness burns, since all these structures are totally destroyed, skin grafting (removing skin from one area of the body and transplanting it to another) is needed for complete healing.

While superficial and partial-thickness burns may be extremely painful, full-thickness burns are usually painless because sensory nerves, that normally carry pain, are destroyed along with the other skin tissues.

Are all burns caused by heat or fire?
No, burns may also be caused by scalding, when a hot liquid comes in contact with the skin. Usually these burns are superficial, or partial-thickness, burns; but full-thickness burns may occur, especially in children, because their skin is thin and delicate.

Electrical injuries are another cause of burns. Electrical burns frequently involve the hands and arms and produce deep penetrating wounds which usually look less severe than they really are. All electrical burns require immediate medical attention.

Chemical burns, due to strong acids and bases or other caustic substances, are also common. Although initially superficial or partial-thickness in extent, these burns may, after first contact, continue to slowly extend into deeper tissues causing more extensive injury.

What are the dangers associated with burns?
Superficial burns are usually uncomplicated and heal quickly and completely, but partial and full-thickness burns are another story. Since dead tissue provides excellent food for bacteria, these burns are prone to infection and frequently become contaminated by millions of growing bacteria within forty-eight hours. If left untreated, the invasion of bacteria will eventually extend deeper and deeper into the underlying areas of the skin, and possibly even gain access to the bloodstream, thus provoking a serious general illness.

There are other major complications associated with severe burns which make physician assistance and hospitalization absolutely necessary. With extensive deep burns, shock, lung congestion, and stomach ulcers frequently occur.

When should burns be self-treated?
Certainly superficial burns can be self-treated since they are generally small and uncomplicated. Limited partial-thickness burns may also be self-treated by conscientious individuals who will take the time to provide themselves with adequate therapy. These burns are characterized by redness, blistering, and superficial skin peeling and should not exceed a few inches in diameter or 30 square inches of total area burned. All other burns should be brought to the attention of the doctor.

What constitutes good treatment for the different kinds of burns?
The treatment of chemical burns differs according to the nature of the causative agent. However, all chemical burns should be immediately neutralized, and the offending substance should be removed as quickly as possible. Acid and alkali burns should be washed thoroughly with large quantities of water. After cleansing, acid burns can be neutralized with sodium bicarbonate and alkali burns can be bathed

with vinegar. Other chemicals require specific methods of removal, so professional advice is wisely sought in these cases.

With electrical burns, the victim's life may depend upon immediate life-support measures because of the devastating effect electricity has on the brain and heart. As I mentioned before, all electrical burns require professional therapy, and immediate measures should be taken to provide that help.

Thermal burns, those resulting from fire or heat, should immediately be cooled with cold water, or ice if it is available; this practice will limit the extent of injury. Apply the water or ice until the pain has subsided or for one hour. If pain returns apply more ice.

Once these initial first aid steps have been performed, treatment should be directed at prevention of infection and relief from pain.

How can infection of a burn be prevented?
After following the first aid measures just described, washing the burned area with a mild solution of soapy water will remove contaminants and reduce the number of bacteria normally present on the skin surface. Once this is done, an antibacterial ointment or cream can be applied, and a patch of gauze can be used to lightly cover the wound.

RECOMMENDED TREATMENT
Since burn infections may be caused by a variety of bacteria, a broad-spectrum antibiotic (one that is effective against many different germs) should be used. Fortunately, there are numerous excellent over-the-counter preparations, which contain one or more broad-spectrum antibiotics that have been proven effective against the bacteria commonly infecting burns. These antibiotics include bacitracin, neomycin, polymyxin, and tetracycline.

COMMENTS AND CAUTIONS
Many products that are marketed for burns can actually be detrimental. Anesthetic creams, lotions, and sprays,

those that contain benzocaine or any of the other "caines," should not be used. These may actually slow the healing process, and, in some unfortunate victims, further irritate or even sensitize already damaged skin. Furthermore, these products do not contain the antibiotics that are needed to prevent secondary bacterial infection. Don't be fooled by the way these products relieve burn pain. The discomfort will quickly return and additional complications may actually prolong your suffering.

ANTIBIOTIC CREAMS AND OINTMENTS
For a listing of these medications, please turn to Chapter 11, "Cuts, Scrapes, and Scratches"(pages 143-44).

7. Colds and Flus

What is a common cold?
The common cold is a viral infection of the upper respiratory tract.

What is the upper respiratory tract?
The upper respiratory tract consists of those passages that carry air to and from the lungs. These include the nose and sinuses, the upper throat, the larynx or voice box, the trachea (an air tube that connects the larynx with the lungs), and the bronchi (the air tubes that extend from the trachea into the lungs).

What is a virus?
A virus is the most simple of all living organisms and is found throughout nature. It is smaller than a bacterium and, like bacteria, can infect humans and cause illnesses. Structurally, viruses consist of a string of genes, DNA or RNA, and a thin protein covering. Both the genes and the surrounding protein differ from one virus to another, making each type of virus specifically different.

How does a person get a cold?
Our surroundings are loaded with millions of bacteria and viruses, some of which cause disease and illness while others have no effect at all. When we are exposed to a sufficient number of cold viruses and they gain entrance into our bodies through the nose or the mouth, we will catch cold if our immunities are insufficient and our natural defenses are

low. If, however, we have had previous exposure to the *same* virus, there is a possibility that our bodies have developed the proper antibodies to fight off the infections. Thus, a person acquires a cold after exposure to an appropriate virus when natural defenses are inadequate.

Are other diseases caused by viruses?
Most certainly! Scientists and doctors have proved that many diseases are caused by viruses, including some forms of cancer. This is not to say that viruses which cause colds also cause cancer. It simply points out that viruses cause many different diseases. Other common diseases produced by viral infections include mumps, measles, and chicken pox, just to name a few.

Is there any prevention for the common cold?
The best way to avoid catching a cold is to stay away from people who have them and from crowded, closed places. People with colds cough, sneeze, and constantly breathe out thousands of viruses contained in microscopic water droplets. To be near an infected person means that you will breathe in these small droplets and allow the viruses contained within them to attack your nose, throat, sinuses, and lungs.

Will vitamin C help to prevent colds?
Much has been written about vitamin C and the common cold; to be sure, there are many opinions. Some people swear by it, other say it does nothing. Within the medical community, mixed views also exist, so evaluation of the controversy becomes quite difficult. Yet, amid the confusion, certain undeniable facts have arisen.

First, vitamin C is absolutely needed for a host of body functions, including the constant maintenance of cells and intracellular substances as well as repair of injured tissues. These two functions alone would tend to prevent colds and aid in rapid recovery.

Second, vitamin C has been shown to improve healing in other viral diseases unrelated to the common cold, thus substantiating its beneficial effects on viral diseases in general.

And, recently, new information has strengthened the role of vitamin C in preventing cancer, urinary tract infections, atherosclerosis, and many other illnesses.

Finally, studies on children have highlighted the cold prevention effect of vitamin C (up to 35 percent reductions) and suggest its use prophylactically.

In the face of all this information, daily vitamin C intake is recommended, not only for cold prevention, but for better general health. How much? At least 500 milligrams daily, although some dietary experts suggest higher doses.

When viruses are present within the upper respiratory tract, what do they do?
Viruses enter the cells that line your nose, throat, larynx, trachea, and bronchi. Once inside these cells, they actually use *your* nutrients and biological processes to reproduce. The new young viruses then break out of these used cells, leaving them injured or dying, and go on to invade additional new cells, multiplying by the same process.

When are common colds spread?
It must always be remembered that colds are relatively mild, yet highly contagious illnesses, occurring mostly indoors and predominantly in the winter months. Actually, three peak cold seasons are identified each year. The first peak occurs a few weeks after schools open in the autumn and undoubtedly reflects the gathering of many children indoors, where a virus may rapidly spread from one ill child to many healthy children. The children then pass the infection to their parents.

The second, and largest, peak is noted in midwinter, when people generally spend more time indoors and when exposure to severe cold weather may itself cause minor changes or slight irritation of the upper respiratory tract. Thus, a virus is allowed to get a foothold.

Finally, a third small peak occurs in the spring.

Who is affected?
Everybody is affected by the common cold. Children, between the ages of one and five, get the most colds. They average about six each year. Young adults may experience three to four colds per year, and older persons generally contract two or three colds annually.

How does the upper respiratory tract change in response to infection?
The following principal changes are associated with a viral infection and cell injury.

Congestion: In an attempt to fight the infection, blood vessels enlarge in response to histamines released at the site of viral invasion. In this way, excessive amounts of blood flow into affected areas. Capillaries, the smallest of blood vessels, then allow increased amounts of fluid to escape from the blood.

Edema: As fluid leaves the capillaries, it collects in the tissue that lines the upper respiratory tract and causes swelling.

Increased mucus: The cells lining the upper respiratory tract produce thin, watery mucus and, when they are affected by viral infection, the production of this mucus increases.

Pain: As swelling increases and nasal sinuses become clogged with secretions, nerves in these areas become stretched, pressurized, and produce pain. Also, viral, chemical, and other physical irritants injure sensitive exposed nerve endings, causing soreness and suffering.

Do these responses cause the symptoms of a common cold?
Yes. The onset of a cold is usually quite rapid. At first, a soreness of the throat is noted, followed in several hours by congestion of the nasal passages and the presence of thin, watery mucus running from the nose. Sneezing may also occur, due to nasal irritation.

Within forty-eight hours, breathing may become difficult,

the sense of taste and smell may diminish, a cough may develop, and the voice may become harsh due to congestion and edema of the vocal cords. Minor aches and pains of muscles and general fatigue occasionally ensue.

In adults, fever is ordinarily absent. However, children frequently run a temperature as high as 103°.

The common cold usually is self-limiting and runs a variable course lasting seven to fourteen days. Congestion of the nasal passages and sinuses along with a slight cough are usually the most persistent symptoms, but these, too, gradually disappear as the illness abates.

Is there a cure for the common cold?
No. There is no cure for the common cold!

Can a cold at least be treated successfully?
Yes. The first step in treating the common cold is to drink plenty of liquids, maintain a good balanced diet, and get plenty of rest. In addition, many excellent products, which bring temporary relief of cold symptoms, can be purchased without a prescription. Medication should be directed at the most bothersome symptoms, not all of the symptoms, and should be discontinued as soon as the illness subsides.

Should a doctor be consulted for a common cold?
Generally not. Colds are simple common ailments that can be self-treated easily and successfully in most cases, saving the doctor's time and your money. If, however, cold symptoms extend beyond the average ten to fourteen days or become increasingly worse instead of better, a physician's intervention is wisely sought. Other complications that should direct you to your doctor include persistent earaches; prolonged fever; pus or blood in your mucus or sputum; persistent sore throat or large swollen glands.

What cold symptoms can be self-treated?
Medication is available over the counter for coughs, nasal and sinus congestion and stuffiness, fever, pain, sore throats, and lung congestion. The treatment of body aches and pains

and fever is covered in chapters 1 and 19 of this book. For the purposes of this chapter, I will cover the treatment of the most common symptoms of the cold: coughs, nasal and sinus congestion, and sore throats.

COUGHS

What causes a cough?
Basically, there are two main causes for a cough. Either the air tubes leading to the lungs become obstructed by phlegm, mucus, or even foreign obstacles that are inadvertently swallowed and inhaled, or they become sore and irritated from infection or inflammation. Both of the above conditions, obstruction and irritation, provoke a reflex that initiates coughing.

Are all coughs bad?
No. When coughing is due to obstruction of air passages, it is actually beneficial and may even be lifesaving. By forcefully blowing a puff of air through the respiratory tract, a cough will clear away the blockage and allow air to flow freely to and from the lungs. Other coughs, those due to irritation rather than blockage, usually are not good and only provoke additional tenderness and soreness.

Should all coughs be suppressed?
No! Productive coughs that promote free breathing by bringing up mucus and phlegm should not be treated. Remember, these are beneficial and maintain a clear passageway to the lungs. Allow them to work. Coughs that are due to rawness from smoking or other forms of irritation, like postnasal drip, and productive coughs which persist, after the air tubes have cleared and become dry, should be treated. They are not beneficial and serve no real purpose except to inform us that the air passages are unhealthy.

Are there different types of cough medicines?
There are two different types of cough medicines. One type is intended for the sole purpose of stopping coughs and should

be used when the cough is dry, hacking, and nonproductive. This is called a suppressant. The second actually *promotes* coughing, and this type is called an expectorant.

What are the active cough ingredients found in cough suppressants?

The following drugs will suppress coughs and are found in most over-the-counter cough medications. Many prescription products contain the same ingredients.

Codeine: Through the years, codeine has been considered to be the most appropriate cough medication available, and that opinion is still widely upheld today. Although an addictive effect is noted when the medication is taken in excessive amounts, proper use of recommended dosages virtually eliminates the possiblity of mental or physical dependence. Generally, codeine therapy is without side effects in both children and adults, although, rarely, constipation, sleepiness, nausea, and itching may occur. Furthermore, codeine should not be taken by people with long-standing lung disease or by individuals who have demonstrated previous allergy to this drug.

Dextromethorphan: This drug has shown effectiveness as a cough preparation but generally is not considered as effective as codeine. Side effects caused by this drug are infrequent, but they include upset stomach and other mild disturbances of the intestines, plus sleepiness. Due to the safety of this medication, it can be taken by almost anyone except people who are allergic to it.

Diphenhydramine: Diphenhydramine is actually an antihistamine which has cough suppressant qualities and has recently received approval as an over-the-counter cough medication. Since this drug is a strong antihistamine, it has a profound sedative effect and may cause drowsiness in some individuals. It should not be taken by people with asthma, glaucoma, or prostate enlargement and should be avoided by patients on tranquilizers, sedatives, hypnotics, anticholinergics, and monoamine oxidase inhibitors. Pregnant women should also avoid it.

Noscapine: This medication, a derivative of opium, is nonaddictive and demonstrates effectiveness as a cough suppressant. Apparently safe and without significant side effects, noscapine is suitable for general use. However, since this drug is relatively new, further studies are under way.

What is an expectorant?
Expectorants are substances which increase the watery secretions normally produced by the cells lining the upper respiratory tract. These watery secretions are useful in loosening thick mucus and phlegm that build up within the lungs during respiratory illnesses. Once the phlegm is watered down, the normal cough reflex will *promote* its removal from the lungs, allowing more normal breathing. Thus, the expectorant does not suppress the cough, it loosens secretions so they can be expelled.

What are the expectorants found in over-the-counter medications?
The variety of expectorants in OTC products are unrelated chemically and have different modes of actions. Serious side effects are noted in some. Their good and bad points are listed below.

Ammonium chloride: Ammonium chloride works by causing a mild irritation of the lining of the stomach which, in turn, triggers a reflex that stimulates the flow of respiratory secretions. This is known as reflex stimulation, and most expectorants in over-the-counter medications work in this manner.

Ammonium chloride can cause serious side effects in people with liver, kidney, or heart disease. Also, if the drug is taken in excess, serious problems can result even in healthy people. Therefore, this drug must be used with caution.

Guaifenesin: This is another expectorant that works by reflex stimulation and thus carries the potential side effect of stomach upset, although this adverse reaction is rare. A more serious complication is this drug's ill effect on the blood components that stop bleeding (platelets), but this apparently only occurs if the drug is taken in excessive quantities.

Ipecac: Another reflex stimulator, ipecac, can be used as

an expectorant and is found in several OTC preparations. This substance is also used to induce vomiting in cases of poisoning by mouth and therefore may cause vomiting when used as an expectorant. Ipecac is not recommended for children under six years of age.

Guaiacolate: Guaiacolate is a reflex stimulator similar to guaifenesin.

Terpin hydrate: Unlike the expectorants previously described, terpin hydrate promotes increased respiratory-tract secretions by a direct stimulating effect on the secretory cells themselves. Therefore, it is less apt to cause stomach discomfort.

NASAL AND SINUS CONGESTION

How do drugs reduce nasal and sinus congestion?
As mentioned previously, one of the symptoms of the common cold is nasal stuffiness caused by the enlargement of blood vessels, increased blood flow to the nasal lining, and swelling of nasal tissue because of fluid collection (edema). Nasal sprays and drops work by stimulating the small blood vessels to reduce in size, thus decreasing blood flow and eliminating edema and swelling. As the engorged membranes lining the nose reduce in size, free breathing is restored, pressure and pain are eliminated, and proper nasal drainage can resume. Nasal and sinus congestion can be treated by using either a nasal spray decongestant or an oral decongestant.

What are the medications available in OTC nasal decongestant products?
Closely related, but varying in potency and duration of action, the following medications are available without a prescription.

Phenylephrine: Phenylephrine is most popular and has long been used as an effective agent for nasal congestion, but its use it not without complications. It may produce a "rebound" effect; that is, when the drug wears off, congestion returns and is more severe than it was before the drug was used. Significant nasal irritation may also occur.

Levodesoxyephedrine: This drug is primarily found in inhalants and works directly on congested blood vessels. Irritation and rebound effect are also noted with this product, and in cases of severe congestion, where air flow through the nose is nil, levodesoxyephedrine may be totally ineffective because inhalants fail to deliver it adequately.

Naphazoline: Probably the most potent of all the nasal decongestants, naphazoline has a moderately long duration of action. Although it is not recommended for children, adults can safely use this product if they follow directions. Stinging may be noted immediately following application, and nasal irritation does occur.

Oxymetazoline and *xylometazoline:* These two drugs are long-acting nasal decongestants with effects that last six hours or more. Rebound is less likely with these products because their effect is long lasting and they can be used less frequently.

Propylhexedrine: Similar to levodesoxyephedrine, propylhexedrine is used in inhalant decongestants. Comparative studies between propylhexedrine and levodesoxyephedrine and the more common nasal decongestants do not exist. Therefore, it is difficult to evaluate the true effectiveness of these two drugs.

When and how should nasal decongestants be used?
When nasal congestion is severe and breathing is difficult, a decongestant is appropriately used. These products come in squeeze-bottle sprays, drop dispensers, and inhalers. If a dropper is used, the proper measured amount (measurement marks are found on the droppers) should be placed in each nostril and sniffed deeply into the nose. Tilting the head backward or lying on your back with your head extending over the side of the bed will facilitate the application. A few minutes should pass before you assume the normal upright position.

Sprays are used by administering one squeeze into each nostril as you again sniff the medication high into your nose. You should then wait a few minutes, blow your nose to remove any excess mucus, and apply a second spray if breathing is still difficult.

What are oral decongestants?

These are products which can be taken by mouth for reducing upper respiratory-tract congestion. Unlike nose drops, sprays, and inhalants, they exert an effect on the entire body because they are absorbed from the stomach and intestines, then carried within the blood stream to all parts of the body. Since they have a particularly strong effect on the blood vessels of the upper respiratory tract, they aid in reducing swelling and congestion there.

What are some of the other effects of oral decongestants?

The oral decongestants may cause slight changes in blood pressure, increase the heart rate, enlarge the air passages of the lungs, cause the heart to beat irregularly, raise the blood sugar, and cause mild nervous stimulation that may lead to irritability and insomnia. Those products that contain antihistamines may also cause drowsiness.

Can anyone use oral decongestants?

The great majority of people can safely take these drugs without any problem. However, diabetics, heart patients, and those individuals who suffer from high blood pressure and thyroid disease should consult a doctor before using these products. Furthermore, they should not be used by patients taking monoamine oxidase inhibitor drugs that are frequently prescribed for depression.

What drugs are used as oral decongestants?

All of the drugs, which follow, are closely related and are used as decongestants.

Ephedrine: Nasal and sinus congestion are reduced by ephedrine, and this drug also produces significant widening of the air passages in the lungs (bronchodilation). Its use is associated with a mild stimulating effect on the nervous system.

Phenylephrine: Described previously under nasal decongestants, this drug can also be taken by mouth, although it is less effective when used in this manner.

Phenylpropanolamine: Similar to ephedrine, but this drug has a greater decongestant effect and less of a bronchodilating action.

Pseudoephedrine: This drug is also similar to ephedrine but less effective. It does not seem to produce as much nervous stimulation either.

When should oral decongestants be taken?
Oral decongestants are useful when difficulty in breathing is associated more with a tightness in the chest and lungs than with a nasal congestion. When necessary, a drug like ephedrine is particularly useful since it not only reduces congestion but also enlarges the air passages of the lung. If nasal congestion is a major problem, I recommend nasal sprays or drops. They are also beneficial in reducing the pain and swelling of sinus congestion and "stuffy ears."

SORE THROATS

Sore throats are very common, but are they very serious?
Most sore throats, at least those caused by cold viruses, are not serious. They cause only temporary discomfort and are usually gone within a few days. Likewise, the acute sore throat associated with smoking is usually insignificant and passes with time. But there are sore throats that are serious. These are caused by the streptococcal bacteria that give rise to the name "strep throat" and can lead to rheumatic fever and its associated kidney, heart, and blood complications—conditions that are truly life threatening. Also, the chronic throat irritation that results from heavy smoking may ultimately progress into throat cancer.

How can you tell the cause of your sore throat?
If you are a smoker and frequently misuse tobacco products, you probably will suffer intermittent sore throats because of your habit. No other sign of illness will be noted.

When the sore throat is present with other symptoms, like a runny nose, sinus congestion, coughing, and sneezing, you most likely have a cold or the flu. And, if the irritation is noticed only in the morning during the winter months when the heater is running, it is usually due to excessive drying of the mucus membranes from the lack of moisture in heated air.

Strep throat, on the other hand, is usually associated with pus around the tonsils and along the back of the throat; this can be seen using a good light and a mirror. Fever, swollen glands, and a skin rash may also be present, and previous strep throats make the diagnosis more likely.

What should you do?
Strep throat must be treated with antibiotics from your doctor as soon as possible. If you suspect strep, have a throat culture performed immediately and begin the necessary physician-directed therapy if that culture is positive.

For those minor sore throat irritations not caused by strep, self-directed treatments are advised. These include saltwater gargles, increased fluid intake, room humidification, and aspirin or aspirin substitutes for discomfort. OTC lozenges may also provide temporary relief from pain. Smoking must be discontinued.

Should sore throats in children be parent-medicated?
Again, if the sore throat is associated with obvious cold symptoms it can be parent-medicated, but it usually need not be. Since the sore throat of a common cold passes quickly, medication is usually unnecessary. Sore throats in children which are not accompanied by other cold symptoms should definitely be brought to the attention of a physician, especially when a rash and fever are present.

What medications are found in over-the-counter sore throat products?
Benzocaine: Benzocaine is an anesthetic which is similar to novocaine in that it temporarily deadens nerves and blocks the sensation of pain.

Benzyl alcohol: Benzyl alcohol is another safe and effective surface anesthetic.

Phenol and *sodium phenolate:* These substances also deaden nerves, but they have the added effect of being antibacterial agents: they kill germs.

RECOMMENDED TREATMENT

COUGHS

Suppressants: Of all the cough suppressants, codeine is the most effective. Unfortunately, many states restrict its over-the-counter sale, making it a prescription item. Check with your pharmacist about this, and ask if you may sign for the codeine you need. Frequently, this procedure is acceptable, although the quantity available on signing is rather limited.

As a alternative, I recommend dextromethorphan. It, too, is very effective and can be purchased anywhere, anytime. Regardless of your choice, be sure to pick the cough suppressant with the fewest number of additional ingredients. Antihistamines should generally be avoided because they dry up secretions which tend to block air passages. And decongestants are unnecessary when the only problem is a cough.

Expectorants: The effectiveness of these drugs has been questioned time and again, and studies set up to determine their worth are inconclusive. As mentioned earlier, because of the possible side effects of ammonium chloride and ipecac, I would not recommend these drugs. Guaifenesin and guaiacolate seem safe enough, and these I would use.

NASAL AND SINUS CONGESTION

Nasal Decongestants: Because of the ease and convenience of nasal sprays, I recommend these products for older children and adults. For younger children, who generally have difficulty with sprays, I suggest nose drops. Of the various OTC medications for nasal congestion, I prefer those that contain oxymetazoline or xylometazoline because of their long-lasting nature and decreased rebound effect. Naphazoline is also acceptable for adults, but remember, irritation of the nasal lining may occur with its use.

Oral Decongestants: The question as to which is the best oral decongestant is open to much debate, and I can only offer my opinion. In my mind, ephedrine and phenylpropanolamine are likely choices.

SORE THROAT

The best products are those that contain an anesthetic agent such as benzocaine, benzyl alcohol, phenol, and sodium phenolate.

COMMENTS AND CAUTIONS

COUGHS

Cough treatment takes many forms. Breathing moist air from a humidifier or shower helps to soothe the irritated lining of the air passages and also loosens sticky, dry secretions. Drinking plenty of fluids helps in this regard as well. Dry, hacking, nonproductive coughs should be suppressed, and congested coughs that produce thick mucus should be treated with an expectorant. Once again, if the cough is productive and has a beneficial effect, let it alone; treat it only if it dries up and becomes irritating.

If your cough is associated with a high or prolonged fever it is best to see your doctor. Also, when coughing produces thick, foul-smelling mucus and pus it probably means you have a bacterial infection of the lungs or bronchial airways. This should be treated with antibiotics and only your doctor can prescribe these adequately.

NASAL AND SINUS CONGESTION

As with any medication, nasal decongestants should only be used in recommended doses at specific time periods as directed by the manufacturer. Medication should cease as soon as the illness or symptom clears.

Problems associated with nasal decongestants are mostly related to their overuse and include nasal irritation and rebound congestion. The person who continuously uses nasal drops and sprays may be treating a problem actually caused by those products. If this is suspected, the use of the nasal spray should be stopped immediately and an oral decongestant may be taken while the previous drug effects wear away, in 2 to 3 days.

Although oral decongestants contain acceptable ingredients, they also incorporate other drugs which need not be taken. For example, many products also contain belladonna (depressant), caffeine (stimulant), alcohol, aspirin, acetaminophen (pain killer), phenacetin (pain killer), and various antihistamines. The oral decongestant that has few of these unneeded drugs but contains either ephedrine or phenylpropanolamine is, in my opinion, the best.

SORE THROAT

Additional substances to the anesthetic agents mentioned above, such as cough suppressants, decongestants, expectorants, and antibacterial compounds are unnecessary in treating the sore throat of a common cold. Therefore, they should be avoided.

COLD MEDICATIONS

Boldface: Recommended

COUGH PREPARATIONS

SUPPRESSANTS/EXPECTORANTS

Actol, liquid

noscapine 30 mg/5 ml
guaifenesin 200 mg/5 ml
alcohol 12.5%

Alamine,
expectorant liquid

codeine phosphate 5 mg/5 ml
guaifenesin 100 mg/5 ml
phenylephrine hydrochloride 10 mg/5 ml
chlorpheniramine maleate 2 mg/5 ml
menthol 1 mg/5 ml
alcohol 5%

Alamine-C, liquid

codeine phosphate 5 mg/5 ml
phenylephrine hydrochloride 10 mg 5 ml
chlorpheniramine maleate 2 mg/5 ml
menthol 1 mg/5 ml
alcohol 5%

Alo-Tuss, tablet

dextromethorphan hydrobromide 10 mg
phenylephrine hydrochloride 5 mg
chlorpheniramine maleate 2 mg

Arrestin, tablet

dextromethorphan hydrobromide 10 mg
guaiacolate 25 mg
alcohol 10%

Atussin D.M.,
expectorant

dextromethorphan hydrobromide 15 mg/
    5ml
guaifenesin 100 mg/5 ml
phenylephrine hydrochloride 5 mg/5 ml
phenylpropanolamine hydrochloride
    5mg/5 ml
chlorpheniramine maleate 2 mg/5 ml

Benylin, liquid

diphenhydramine hydrochloride 12.5 mg/
    5 ml

Breacol, liquid

dextromethorphan hydrobromide 10 mg/
   5 ml
phenylpropanolamine hydrochloride
   37.5 mg/5 ml
chlorpheniramine maleate 4 mg/5 ml
alcohol 10%

Broncho-Tussin,
liquid

codeine phosphate 65 mg/30 ml
potassium guaiacolsulfonate 520 mg/30
ml
terpin hydrate 260 mg/30 ml
ammonium hypophosphite 520 mg/30 ml
alcohol 40%

C 3 Capsules

dextromethorphan hydrobromide 30 mg
phenylpropanolamine hydrochloride
   50 mg
chlorpheniramine maleate 5 mg

Cerose DM, liquid

dextromethorphan hydrobromide 10 mg/
   5 ml
potassium guaiacolsulfonate 86 mg/5 ml
ipecac fluid extract 0.17 min/5 ml
phenylephrine hydrochloride 5 mg/5 ml
phenindamine tartrate 5 mg/5 ml
sodium citrate 195 mg/5 ml
citric acid 65 mg/5 ml
glycerin 40 min/5 ml
alcohol 2.5%

Cheracol, liquid

codeine phosphate 10 mg/5 ml
guaifenesin 100 mg/5 ml
alcohol 3%

Cheracol D, liquid

dextromethorphan hydrobromide 10 mg/
   5 ml
guaifenesin 15 mg/5 ml
alcohol 3%

Chlor-Trimeton
Expectorant with
Codeine, liquid

codeine 10 mg/5 ml
ammonium chloride 100 mg/5 ml
guaifenesin 50 mg/5 ml
phenylephrine hydrochloride 10 mg/5 ml
chlorpheniramine maleate 2 mg/5 ml
sodium citrate 50 mg/5 ml
alcohol 1%

Cidicol, liquid

ethylmorphine hydrochloride 16.25 mg/
  30 ml
potassium guaiacolsulfonate 520 mg/
  30 ml
alcohol 5%
potassium citrate
citric acid

Codimal DM, liquid

dextromethorphan hydrobromide 10 mg/
  5 ml
potassium guaiacolsulfonate 83.3 mg/5 ml
phenylephrine hydrochloride 5 mg/5 ml
pyrilamine maleate 8.33 mg/5 ml
sodium citrate 216 mg/5 ml
citric acid 50 mg/5 ml
alcohol 5%

Codimal PH, liquid

codeine phosphate 10 mg/5 ml
potassium guaiacolsulfonate 83.3 mg/5 ml
phenylephrine hydrochloride 5 mg/5 ml
pyrilamine maleate 8.33 mg/5 ml
sodium citrate 216 mg/5 ml
citric acid 50 mg/5 ml

Cold Team
Nighttime, liquid

dextromethorpan hydrobromide 15 mg/
  5 ml
phenylephrine hydrochloride 5 mg/5 ml
chlorpheniramine maleate 1 mg/5 ml

Colrex, liquid

dextromethorphan hydrobromide 10 mg/
  5 ml
potassium guaiacolsulfonate 80 mg/5 ml
ammonium chloride 80 mg/5 ml
phenylephrine hydrochloride 5 mg/5 ml
chlorpheniramine maleate 1 mg/5 ml

Conar, liquid

noscapine 15 mg/5 ml
phenylephrine hydrochloride 10 mg/5 ml

Conar, expectorant
liquid

noscapine 15 mg/5 ml
guaifenesin 100 mg/5 ml
phenylephrine hydrochloride 10 mg/5 ml

Conex W-Codeine, liquid — codeine phosphate 10 mg/10 ml
guaifenesin 50 mg/10 ml
phenylpropanolamine hydrochloride
   25 mg/10 ml
chlorpheniramine maleate 2 mg/10 ml
methylparaben 0.13%
propylparaben 0.03%

Congesprin Cough Syrup for Children — dextromethorphan hydrobromide 5 mg/
   5 ml

Consotuss, liquid — dextromethorphan hydrobromide 15 mg/
   5 ml
doxylamine succinate 3.75 mg/5 ml
alcohol 10%

Contac Jr., liquid — dextromethorphan hydrobromide 5 mg/
   5 ml
phenylpropanolamine hydrochloride
   0.375 mg/5 ml
acetaminophen 162.5 mg/5 ml
alcohol 10%

Coryban-D, liquid — dextromethorphan hydrobromide 7.5 mg/
   5 ml
guaifenesin 50 mg/5 ml
phenylephrine hydrocholoride 5 mg/5 ml
alcohol 7.5%
acetaminophen 120 mg/5 ml

C., liquid — Vitamin C 12.5 mg/5 ml

Cosanyl DM Improved Formula, liquid — dextromethorphan hydrobromide 15 mg/
   5 ml
pseudoephedrine hydrochloride 30 mg/
   5 ml
alcohol 6%

Cough Syrup for Children — dextromethorphan hydrobromide 7.5 mg
phenylpropanolamine hydrochloride 9 mg
alcohol 5%

DayCare, liquid — dextromethorphan hydrobromide 20 mg/
   30 ml
phenylpropanolamine hydrochloride
   25 mg/30 ml
acetaminophen 600 mg/30 ml

Dimocol, liquid	dextromethorphan hydrobromide 15 mg/
	    5 ml
	guaifenesin 100 mg/5 ml
	pseudoephedrine hydrochloride 30 mg/
	    5 ml
	alcohol 4.75%

Dimocol, capsule	dextromethorphan hydrobromide 15 mg guaifenesin 100 mg pseudoephedrine hydrochloride 30 mg
DM–4 Children's Cough Control, liquid	dextromethorphan hydrobromide 4 mg/ 5 ml ammonium chloride 50 mg/5 ml potassium guaiacolsulfonate 38 mg/5 ml glycerin 75 mg/5 ml alcohol 1.5%
DM–8, liquid	dextromethorphan hydrobromide 8 mg/ 5 ml ammonium chloride 80 mg/5 ml potassium guaiacolsulfonate 75 mg/5 ml alcohol 3%
Dondril Anticough, tablet	dextromethorphan hydrobromide 10 mg guaifenesin 50 mg phenylephrine hydrochloride 5 mg chlorpheniramine maleate 1 mg

Dorcol Pediatric,
liquid
	dextromethorphan hydrobromide 7.5 mg/
	    5 ml
	guaifenesin 37.5 mg/5 ml
	phenylpropanolamine hydrochloride
	    8.75 mg/5 ml
	alcohol 5%

Dristan, liquid	dextromethorphan hydrobromide 7.5 mg/ 5 ml phenylephrine hydrochloride 5 mg/5 ml chlorpheniramine maleate 1 mg/5 ml sodium citrate alcohol 12%
Duad, capsule	dextromethorphan hydrobromide 10 mg sodium citrate 50 mg benzocaine 3 mg

Efricon, liquid — codeine phosphate 10.96 mg/5 ml
ammonium chloride 90 mg/5 ml
potassium guaiacolsulfonate 90 mg/5 ml
phenylephrine hydrochloride 5 mg/5 ml
chlorpheniramine maleate 2 mg/5 ml
sodium citrate 60 mg/5 ml

Endotussin NN, liquid — dextromethorphan hydrobromide 10 mg/ 5 ml
ammonium chloride 50 mg/5 ml
pyrilamine maleate 7.5 mg/5 ml
homatropine methylbromide 0.25 mg/ 5 ml

Endotussin NN Pediatric, liquid — dextromethorphan hydrobromide 5 mg/ 1 ml
ammonium chloride 60 mg/1 ml
homatropine methylbromide 0.15 mg/ 1 ml

Formula 44, disc — dextromethorphan hydrobromide 10 mg
doxylamine succinate 6 mg
sodium citrate 500 mg
alcohol 10%

2/G-DM, liquid — dextromethorphan hydrobromide 15 mg/ 5 ml
guaifenesin 100 mg/5 ml
alcohol 5%
corn derivatives

Halls, liquid — dextromethorphan hydrobromide 15 mg/ 10 ml
phenylpropanolamine hydrochloride 37.5 mg/10 ml
menthol
eucalyptus oil
alcohol 22%
glycerin

Histadyl EC, liquid — codeine phosphate 64.8 mg/30 ml
ammonium chloride 660 mg/30 ml
ephedrine hydrochloride 30 mg/30 ml
methapyrilene fumarate 81 mg/30 ml
menthol
alcohol 5%

Histivite-D, liquid

dextromethorphan hydrobromide 30 mg/
   30 ml
ammonium chloride 518 mg/30 ml
ephedrine sulfate 24.3 mg/30 ml
methapyrilene fumarate 75 mg/30 ml
menthol
alcohol 4.8%

Kleer Chewable
Tablets

dextromethorphan hydrobromide 2.5 mg
phenylephrine hydrochloride 5 mg
chlorpheniramine maleate 2 mg

Listerine Big 4,
liquid

dextromethorphan hydrobromide
   3.25 mg/5 ml
phenylpropanolamine hydrochloride
   8.5 mg/5 ml
chlorpheniramine maleate 0.5 mg/5 ml
guaiacolate 25 mg/5 ml

Mercodal, liquid

codeine phosphate 10 mg
etafedrine hydrochloride 10 mg
phenylephrine hydrochloride 5 mg
doxylamine succinate 5 mg
alcohol 5 mg

Minituss, liquid

dextromethorphan hydrobromide 7.5 mg
guaifenesin 100 mg
pseudoephedrine hydrochloride 30 mg
alcohol 5%

Moratuss, liquid

codeine phosphate 20 mg/30 ml
ammonium chloride 195.5 mg/30 ml
potassium guaiacolsulfonate 32.5 mg/
   30 ml
terpin hydrate 32.4 mg/30 ml
cocillana extract 26.6 mg/30 ml
sodium benzoate 0.1%

Naldetuss, liquid

dextromethorphan hydrobromide 15mg/
   5 ml
phenylpropanolamine hydrochloride
   17.5 mg/5 ml
phenyltoloxamine citrate 7.5 mg/5 ml
acetaminophen 162 mg/4 ml

Novahistine DH, liquid
codeine phosphate 10 mg/5 ml
phenylpropanolamine hydrochloride
  18.75 mg/5 ml
alchohol 5%

Novahistine DMX, liquid
dextromethorphan hydrobromide 10 mg/
  5 ml
guaifenesin 100 mg/5 ml
pseudoephedrine hydrochloride 30 mg/
  5 ml
alcohol 70%

Novahistine, expectorant, liquid
codeine phosphate 10 mg/5 ml
guaifenesin 100 mg/5 ml
phenylpropanolamine hydrochloride
  18.75 mg/5 ml
alcohol 7.5%

Nyquil, liquid
dextromethorphan hydrobromide 15 mg/
  30 ml
ephedrine sulfate 8 mg/30 ml
doxylamine succinate 7.5 mg/30 ml
acetaminopen 600 mg/30 ml
alcohol 25%

Ornacol, capsule
dextromethorphan hydrobromide 30 mg
phenylpropanolamine hydrochloride
  25 mg

Ornacol, liquid
dextromethorphan hydrobromide 15 mg/
  5 ml
phenylpropanolamine hydrochloride
  12.5 mg/5 ml
alcohol 8%

Orthoxicol, liquid
dextromethorphan hydrobromide 10 mg/
  5 ml
methoxyphenamine hydrochloride 17 mg/
  5 ml

Pertussin 8-hour, liquid
dextromethorphan hydrobromide 30 mg/
  20 ml
alcohol 9.5%

Pertussin Wild
Berry, liquid

dextromethorphan hydrobromide 15 mg/
   20 ml
guaifenesin 100 mg/20 ml
alcohol 8.5%

Prunicodeine, liquid

codeine sulfate 65 mg/30 ml
terpin hydrate 175 mg/30 ml
wild cherry
white pine
sanguinaria
alcohol

Quelidrine, liquid

dextromethorphan hydrobromide 10 mg/
   5 ml
ammonium chloride 50 mg/5 ml
ipecac fluid extract 0.005 ml/5 ml
ephedrine hydrochloride 5 mg/5 ml
phenylephrine hydrochloride 5 mg/5 ml
chlorpheniramine maleate 2 mg/5 ml
alcohol 2%

Queltuss, tablet

dextromethorphan hydrobromide 15 mg
guaifenesin 100 mg

Quiet-Nite, liquid

dextromethorphan hydrobromide 15 mg/
   30 ml
ephedrine sulfate 10 mg/30 ml
chlorpheniramine maleate 2 mg/30 ml
acetaminophen 600 mg/30 ml
alcohol 25%

Rhinex, tablet

dextromethorphan 7.5 mg
guaifenesin 50 mg
phenylpropanolamine 12.5 mg
chlorpheniramine maleate 1 mg
ammonium hydrochloride 100 mg
alcohol 5%
chloroform 0.2%

**Robitussin A-CV,
liquid**

codeine phosphate 10 mg/5 ml
guaifenesin 100 mg/5 ml
alcohol 3.5%

Robitussin-CF,
liquid

dextromethorphan hydrobromide 10 mg/
   5 ml
guaifenesin 50 mg/5 ml
phenylpropanolamine hydrochloride
   12.5 mg/5 ml
alcohol 1.4%

**Robitussin-DM,
liquid**

dextromethorphan hydrobromide 15 mg/
   5 ml
guaifenesin 100 mg/5 ml
alcohol 1.4%

Romex, liquid

destromethorphan hydrobromide 10 mg/
   5 ml
guaifenesin 33 mg/5 ml
phenylephrine hydrochloride 5 mg/5 ml
chlorpheniramine maleate/1 mg/5 ml

Romilar III, syrup

dextromethorphan hydrobromide 5 mg/
   5 ml
guaifenesin 50 mg/5 ml
phenylpropanolamine hydrochloride
   12.5 mg/5 ml
alcohol 10%

Romilar, capsule

dextromethorphan hydrobromide 15 mg
phenylephrine hydrochloride 5 mg
chlorpheniramine maleate 1 mg
acetaminophen 120 mg

Romilar CF, syrup

dextromethorphan hydrobromide 15 mg/
   5 ml
chlorpheniramine maleate 1 mg/5 ml
acetaminophen 120 mg/5 ml
alcohol 10%

**Romilar Chewable
Tablets for
Children**

dextromethorphan hydrobromide 7.5 mg
benzocaine 2 mg

Romilar Children's,
syrup

dextromethorphan hydrobromide 7.5 mg/
   5 ml
guaifenesin 25 mg/5 ml
sodium citrate
citric acid

Silence is Golden, syrup	dextromethorphan hydrobromide 10 mg/ 5 ml
Silexin Cough Syrup	dextromethorphan hydrobromide guaifenesin
Silexin Cough Tablets	dextromethorphan hydrobromide benzocaine
Sorbutuss, syrup	dextromethorphan hydrobromide 10 mg/ 5 ml guaifenesin 100 mg/5 ml ipecac fluid extract 0.003 ml/5 ml potassium citrate 85 mg/5 ml citric acid 35 mg/5 ml glycerin sorbitol vehicle
St. Joseph Cough Syrup for Children	dextromethorphan hydrobromide 7.5 mg/ 5 ml sodium citrate menthol alcohol 0.38%
Supercitin, syrup	dextromethorphan hydrobromide 20 mg/ 10 ml chlorpheniramine maleate 2 mg/10 ml acetaminophen 120 mg/10 ml sodium citrate 100 mg/10 ml
Toclonol, expectorant	carbetapentane citrate 7.25 mg/5 ml terpin hydrate 16.65 mg/5 ml sodium citrate 66.15 mg/5 ml citric acid 6.65 mg/5 ml glycerin 2.8 ml/5 ml menthol 0.83 mg/5 ml alcohol 7.2%
Toclonol with Codeine, expectorant	codeine 10 mg/5 ml carbetapentane citrate 7.25 mg/5 ml terpin hydrate 16.65 mg/5 ml sodium citrate 66.15 mg/5 ml citric acid 6.65 mg/5 ml glycerin 2.8 ml/5 ml menthol 0.83 mg/5 ml alcohol 7.2%

Tolu-Sed, elixir

codeine phosphate 65 mg/30 ml
guaifenesin 600 mg/30 ml
chlorpheniramine maleate 6 mg/30 ml
alcohol 10%

Tolu-Sed DM, elixir

dextromethorphan hydrobromide 10 mg/
    5 ml
guaifenesin 100 mg/5 ml
chlorpheniramine maleate 1 mg/5 ml

Tonecol, syrup

dextromethorphan hydrobromide 10 mg/
    5 ml
guaifenesin 25 mg/5 ml
phenylephrine hydrochloride 5 mg/5 ml
chlorpheniramine maleate 1 mg/5 ml
sodium citrate 15 mg/5 ml
alcohol 7%

Triaminic
Expectorant with
Codeine

codeine phosphate 10 mg/5 ml
guaifenesin 100 mg/5 ml
phenylpropanolamine hydrochloride
    12.5 mg/5 ml
pheniramine maleate 6.25 mg/5 ml
pyrilamine maleate 6.25 mg/5 ml
alcohol 5%

Triaminicol, syrup

dextromethorphan hydrobromide 15 mg/
    5 ml
ammonium chloride 90 mg/5 ml
phenylpropanolamine hydrochloride
    12.5 mg/5 ml
pheniramine maleate 6.25 mg/5 ml
pyrilamine maleate 6.25 mg/5 ml

Trind-DM, syrup

dextromethorphan hydrobromide 7.5 mg/
    5 ml
guaifenesin 50 mg/5 ml
phenylephrine hydrochloride 5 mg/5 ml
acetaminophen 120 mg/5 ml
alcohol 15%

Troutman's, syrup

dextromethorphan hydrochloride 10 mg/
    5 ml
ammonium chloride
alcohol
corn syrup

sucrose
caramel
horehound
menthol
peppermint

Tussagesic   dextromethorphan hydrobromide 15 mg/
Suspension   5 ml
                        terpin hydrate 90 mg/5 ml
                        phenylpropanolamine hydrochloride
                            12.5 mg/5 ml
                        pheniramine maleate 6.25 mg/5 ml
                        pyrilamine maleate 6.25 mg/5 ml
                        acetaminophen 120 mg/5 ml

Tussagesic, tablet   dextromethorphan hydrobromide 30 mg
                        terpin hydrate 180 mg
                        phenylpropanolamine hydrochloride
                            25 mg
                        pheniramine maleate 12.5 mg
                        pyrilamine maleate 12.5 mg
                        acetaminophen 325 mg

Tussar-2, liquid   codeine phosphate 10 mg/5 ml
                        carbetapentane citrate 7.5 mg/5 ml
                        guaifenesin 50 mg/5 ml
                        chlorpheniramine maleate 2.0 mg/5 ml
                        sodium citrate 130 mg/5 ml
                        citric acid 20 mg/5 ml
                        methylparaben 0.1%
                        alcohol 5%

Tussar-SF, liquid   codeine phosphate 10 mg/5 ml
                        carbetapentane citrate 7.5 mg/5 ml
                        guaifenesin 50 mg/5 ml
                        chlorpheniramine maleate 2.0 mg/5 ml
                        sodium citrate 130 mg/5 ml
                        citric acid 20 mg/5 ml
                        methylparaben 0.1%
                        alcohol 12%

Tusscapine, liquid   noscapine 15 mg/5 ml

Vicks, liquid	dextromethorphan hydrobromide 3.5 mg/ 5 ml guaifenesin 25 mg/5 ml sodium citrate 200 mg/5 ml alcohol 5%

EXPECTORANTS

Amonidrin, tablets	ammonium chloride 200 mg guaifenesin 100 mg
Atussin, expectorant liquid	guaifenesin 100 mg/5 ml phenylpropanolamine hydrochloride 5 mg/5 ml phenylephrine hydrochloride 5 ml/5 ml chlorpheniramine maleate 2 mg/5 ml
Baby Cough Syrup	ammonium chloride 13 mg/5 ml glycerin 343 mg/5 ml licorice extract 12 mg/5 ml
Calcidin, tablet	calcium iodide calcium iodate starch
Chlor-Trimeton, expectorant, liquid	ammonium chloride 100 mg/5 ml guaifenesin 50 mg/5 ml phenylephrine hydrochloride 10 mg/5 ml chlorpheniramine maleate 2 mg/5 ml sodium citrate 50 mg/5 ml alcohol 1%
Codimal, expectorant, liquid	potassium guaiacolsulfonate 100 mg/5 ml phenylpropanolamine hydrochloride 25 mg/5 ml sodium citrate 216 mg/5 ml citric acid 50 mg/5 ml
Colrex, expectorant, liquid	guaifenesin 100 mg/5 ml ammonium chloride 50 mg/5 ml alcohol 4.7%

Conex, liquid	guaifenesin 50 mg/10 ml phenylpropanolamine hydrochloride 25 mg/10 ml chlorpheniramine maleate 2 mg/10 ml methylparaben 0.13% propylparaben 0.03%
Coricidin, liquid	ammonium chloride 100 mg/5 ml guaifenesin 50 mg/5 ml phenylpropanolamine hydrochloride 12.5 mg/5 ml chlorpheniramine maleate 2 mg/5 ml
Creomulsion, liquid	creosote ipecac beechwood white pine menthol cascara alcohol
Creo-Terpin, liquid	creosote 133 mg/30 ml terpin hydrate 131 mg/30 ml sodium glycerophosphate 265 mg/30 ml alcohol 25%
Dr. Drake's, liquid	ipecac fluid extract castor oil
Fedahist, expectorant, liquid	guaifenesin 100 mg/5 ml pseudoephedrine hydrochloride 30 mg/ 5 ml chlorpheniramine maleate 2 mg/5 ml
2/G, liquid	guaifenesin 100 mg/5 ml alcohol 3.5% corn derivatives
GG-Cen, capsule	guaifenesin 200 mg
GG-Cen, syrup	guaifenesin 100 mg/5 ml alcohol 10%
GG-Tussin, liquid	guaifenesin 100 mg/3 ml alcohol 3.5%

Hytuss, tablet   guaifenesin 100 mg

Hytuss 2X, capsule   guaifenesin 200 mg

Kiddies Pediatric,   potassium guaiacolsulfonate
liquid   ammonium chloride
                            cocillana extract
                            menthol
                            alcohol 2%

Lanatuss, liquid   guaifenesin 100 mg/5 ml
                            phenylpropanolamine hydrochloride
                                5 mg/5 ml
                            chlorpheniramine maleate 2 mg/5 ml
                            sodium citrate 197 mg/5 ml
                            citric acid 60 mg/5 ml

Neophiban, tablet   guaifenesin 50 mg
                            phenylpropanolamine hydrochloride
                                12.5 mg
                            phenyltoloxamine citrate 25 mg
                            acetaminophen 195 mg

Nortussin, liquid   guaifenesin 100 mg/30 ml
                            alcohol 3.5%

Pediaquil   potassium guaiacolsulfonate 389 mg/
                                30 ml
                            phenylephrine hydrochloride 15 mg/30 ml
                            squill 105 mg/30 ml
                            sorbitol
                            corn syrup

Pinex, liquid   potassium guaiacolsulfonate
                            pine oil
                            eucalyptus oil
                            grindelia extract
                            glycerin

Rem, liquid   ammonium chloride 0.7%
                            ipecac 0.07%
                            alcohol 1.2%
                            white pine 0.47%
                            squill 0.14%
                            lobelia 0.08%

horehound 0.08%
sanguinaria 0.07%
tar 0.07%
menthol 0.05%
tolu 0.004%

Rhinspec, tablet

guaifenesin 100 mg
phenylephrine hydrochloride 5 mg
acetaminophen 300 mg

Robitussin, liquid

guaifenesin 100 mg/5 ml
alcohol 3.5%

Robitussin-PE

guaifenesin 100 mg/5 ml
pseudoephedrine hydrochloride 30 mg/
  5 ml
alcohol 1.4%

**Ryna-Tussadine
Expectorant,
liquid**

guaifenesin 100 mg/5 ml
phenylpropanolamine hydrochloride
  6.25 mg/5 ml
phenylephrine hydrochloride 3.75 mg/
  5 ml
chlorpheniramine maleate 1 mg/5 ml
alcohol 3%

**Ryna-Tussadine
Expectorant,
tablet**

guaifenesin 100 mg
phenylpropanolamine hydrochloride
  6.25 mg
phenylephrine hydrochloride 3.75 mg
pyrilamine maleate 6.25 mg
chlorpheniramine maleate 1 mg

Soltice, liquid

ammonium chloride 170 mg/10 ml
phenylpropanolamine hydrochloride
  25 mg/10 ml
sodium citrate 170 mg/10 ml
cetylpyridinium chloride 0.10 mg/10 ml

**Triaminic,
expectorant, liquid**

guaifenesin 100 mg/5 ml
phenylpropanolamine hydrochloride
  12.5 mg/5 ml
pheniramine maleate 6.15 mg/5 ml
pyrilamine maleate 6.25 mg/5 ml
alcohol 5%

Trind, liquid guaifenesin 50 mg/5 ml
phenylephrine hydrochloride 2.5 mg/5 ml
acetaminophen 120 mg/5 ml
alcohol 15%

Tussciden, guaifenesin 100 mg/5 ml
expectorant, liquid

DECONGESTANTS

TOPICAL (NASAL)

Afrin, nasal spray, oxymetazoline hydrochloride 0.5 mg/1 ml
nose drops benzalkonium chloride 0.2 mg/1 ml
phenylmercuric acetate 0.02 mg/1 ml
sorbitol 40 mg/1 ml
glycine 3.8 mg/1 ml
sodium hydroxide

Alconefrin, nose phenylephrine hydrochloride
drops

Allerest, nasal spray phenylephrine hydrochloride 0.5%
benzalkonium chloride
edetate disodium
sodium bisulfite
saline phosphate buffer

Benzedrex, inhaler propylhexedrine 250 mg

Biomydrin, nasal phenylephrine hydrochloride 0.25%
spray thonzonium bromide 0.05%

Contac Nasal Mist phenylephrine hydrochloride 0.5%
cetylpyridinium chloride 0.02%
thimerosal 0.011%
methapyrilene hydrochloride 0.2%

Coricidin, nasal phenylephrine hydrochloride 5 mg/1 ml
spray

Coryban-D, nasal phenylephrine hydrochloride 0.5%
spray benzalkonium chloride 0.02%

Dristan, inhaler	propylhexedrine menthol eucalyptol methyl salicylate
Dristan, nasal mist	phenylephrine hydrochloride benzalkonium chloride pheniramine maleate menthol eucalyptol methyl salicylate
Duration, nasal spray	oxymetazoline hydrochloride 0.05%
Forthane, inhaler	methylhexaneamine 250 mg menthol 32 mg
Hydra, nasal spray	phenylephrine hydrochloride 0.25% cetyltrimethylammonium bromide 0.25% chlorobutanol 0.25% methapyrilene hydrochloride 0.20%
I-Sedrin Plain, nose drops	ephedrine sulfate 1% chlorobutanol 0.5% gluconic acid
Isophrin Hydrochloride, nasal spray, nose drops	phenylephrine hydrochloride 0.125%; 0.25%; 0.5%; or 1.0%
Naso Mist	phenylephrine hydrochloride 0.5% benzalkonium chloride 0.02% methapyrilene hydrochloride 0.15%
Neo-Synephrine, Hydrochloride, nasal spray	phenylephrine hydrochloride 0.25% and 0.5% benzalkonium chloride 0.02% methyl salicylate menthol camphor eucalyptol
Neo-Synephrine, Hydrochloride, nose drops	phenylephrine hydrochloride 0.125%; 0.25%; 0.5%; and 1.0%

Neo-Synephrine, Hydrochloride, nasal jelly

phenylephrine hydrochloride 0.5%

NTZ, nasal spray, nose drops

phenylephrine hydrochloride 0.5%
benzalkonium chloride 1:5,000
thenyldiamine hydrochloride 0.1%

Privine, nasal spray, nose drops

naphazoline hydrochloride 0.05%
benzalkonium chloride 1:5,000

Pyracort-D, spray

phenylephrine hydrochloride 0.5%

Pyradyne, spray

phenylephrine hydrochloride 0.25%
methapyrilene hydrochloride 0.20%

*Sine-Off Once-A-Day, nasal spray

xylometazoline hydrochloride 0.1%
menthol
eucalyptol
camphor
methyl salicylate

Sinex-LA, nasal spray

xylometazoline hydrochloride 0.1%
thimerosal 0.001%

Sinutab, nasal spray

phenylephrine hydrochloride 0.5%
thonzonium bromide 0.05%

Soltice, nasal spray

phenylephrine hydrochloride 2.6 mg/
   100 ml
methapyrilene hydrochloride 600 mg/
   100 ml

Super Anahist, nasal spray

phenylephrine hydrochloride 0.25%
thimerosal 0.002%
alcohol 0.038%

Triaminicin, nasal spray

phenylpropanolamine hydrochloride
   0.75%
phenylephrine hydrochloride 0.25%
benzalkonium chloride 1:10,000
pheniramine maleate 0.125%
pyrilamine maleate 0.125%

Tuamine, inhaler

tuaminoheptane (equib.) 325 mg
menthol 32 mg

Tyrohist, nasal spray	phenylephrine hydrochloride 0.25% cetalkonium chloride 0.04% pyrilamine maleate 0.15%
Va-Tro-Nol, nose drops	ephedrine sulfate 0.35% thimerosal 0.001% methapyrilene hydrochloride 0.15% menthol eucalyptol camphor methyl salicylate
Vicks, inhaler	levodesoxyephedrine 50 mg menthol camphor methyl salicylate vornyl acetate
Vicks Sinex, nasal spray	phenylephrine hydrochloride 0.50% cetylpyridinium chloride 0.04% thimerosal 0.001% mcthapyrilene hydrochloride 0.12% menthol eucalyptol camphor methyl salicylate
4–Way, nasal spray	phenylephrine hydrochloride 0.05% naphazoline hydrochloride 0.05% phenylpropanolamine hydrochloride 0.2% pyrilamine maleate 0.2%

ORAL

Absinol, tablet	phenylephrine hydrochloride 2.5 mg phenyltoloxamine dihydrogen citrate 25 mg acetaminophen 150 mg salicylamide 150 mg
Alka-Seltzer Plus, effervescent tablet	phenylpropanolamine bitartrate 26.5 mg chlorpheniramine maleate 2.1 mg aspirin 324 mg

Allerest, time capsule
phenylpropanolamine hydrochloride
50 mg
pyrilamine maleate 15 mg
methapyrilene fumarate 10 mg

Allerest Regular, tablet
phenylpropanolamine hydrochloride
18.7 mg
chlorpheniramine maleate 2 mg

Allerest Children's Tablet
phenylpropanolamine hydrochloride
9.4 mg
chlorpheniramine maleate 1 mg

Allergesic, tablet
phenylpropanolamine hydrochloride
25 mg
methapyrilene fumarate 10 mg
chlorpheniramine maleate 1 mg

Allerstat, capsule
phenylpropanolamine 25 mg
phenylephrine hydrochloride 2.5 mg
pheniramine maleate 12.5 mg
pyrilamine maleate 12.5 mg

Alumadrine, tablet
phenylpropanolamine 25 mg
chlorpheniramine maleate 4 mg
acetaminophen 500 mg

Anodynos Forte, tablet
phenylephrine hydrochloride 10 mg
chlorpheniramine maleate 2 mg
salicylamide
acetaminophen
caffeine

Apcohist Allergy, tablet
phenylpropanolamine hydrochloride
25 mg
methapyrilene fumarate 5 mg
chlorpheniramine maleate 1 mg

ARM Allergy Relief Medicine
chlorpheniramine maleate 4 mg
phenylpropanolamine hydrochloride
25 mg

Bayer Children's Cold Tablets
phenylpropanolamine hydrochloride
3.125 mg
aspirin 81 mg

Bayer Decongestant, tablet	phenylpropanolamine hydrochloride 18.75 mg chlorpheniramine maleate 2 mg aspirin 325 mg
BC All Clear, tablet	phenylephrine maleate 10 mg chlorpheniramine maleate 2 mg aspirin 645 mg salicylamide 195 mg caffeine 32 mg cellulose povidone
Benzedrex, inhaler	propylhexedrine 250 mg menthol 12.5 mg aromatics
BQ 6, tablet	quinine hydrobromide 25 mg acetaminophen 100 mg salicylamide 200 mg phenylephrine hydrochloride 5 mg caffeine 15 mg yellow phenolphthalein 10 mg
Cenagesic, tablet	phenylephrine hydrochloride 5 mg pyrilamine maleate 12 mg salicylamide 250 mg phenacetin 120 mg ascorbic acid 30 mg caffeine 15 mg
Chlor-Trimeton, allergy tablets	chlorpheniramine maleate 4 mg
Chlor-Trimeton Decongestant, tablet	ephedrine sulfate 60 mg chlorpheniramine maleate 5 mg
Codimal, tablet, capsule	pseudoephedrine hydrochloride 30 mg chlorpheniramine maleate 2 mg acetaminophen 150 mg salicylamide 150 mg
Colrex, capsule	phenylephrine hydrochloride 5 mg chlorpheniramine maleate 2 mg acetaminophen 300 mg ascorbic acid 200 mg

Conex DA, tablet
phenylpropanolamine hydrochloride 50 mg
phenyltoloxamine citrate 50 mg

Conex Plus, tablet
phenylpropanolamine hydrochloride 25 mg
phenyltoloxamine citrate 25 mg
acetaminophen 250 mg

Congespirin, chewable tablet
phenylephrine hydrochloride 1.25 mg
aspirin 81 mg

Contac, time capsule
phenylpropanolamine hydrochloride 50 mg
chlorpheniramine maleate 5 mg
belladonna alkaloids 0.2 mg

Coricidin, tablet
chlorpheniramine maleate 2 mg
aspirin 325 mg

Coricidin "D," tablet
phenylpropanolamine hydrochloride 12.5 mg
chlorpheniramine maleate 2 mg
aspirin 325 mg

Coricidin Demilets, children's chewable tablet
phenylephrine hydrochloride 2.5 mg
chlorpheniramine maleate 0.5 mg
aspirin 80 mg

Coricidin Medilets, children's chewable tablet
chlorpheniramine maleate 0.5 mg
aspirin 80 mg

Coryban-D, capsule
phenylpropanolamine hydrochloride 25 mg
chlorpheniramine maleate 2 mg
caffeine 30 mg

Co Tylenol, tablet
pseudoephedrine hydrochloride 30 mg
chlorpheniramine maleate 1 mg
acetaminophen 325 mg

Co Tylenol Cold Formula for Children, liquid
pseudoephedrine hydrochloride 7.5 mg/ 5 ml
chlorpheniramine maleate 0.5 mg/5 ml
acetaminophen 120 mg/5 ml
alcohol 7%

Covanamine, liquid	phenylpropanolamine hydrochloride 6.25 mg/5 ml phenylephrine hydrochloride 3.75 mg/ 5 ml pyrilamine maleate 6.25 mg/5 ml chlorpheniramine maleate 1 mg/5 ml
Covangesic, liquid	phenylpropanolamine hydrochloride 6.25 mg. 5 ml phenylephrine hydrochloride 3.75 mg/ 5 ml pyrilamine maleate 6.25 mg/5 ml chlorpheniramine maleate 1.0 mg/5 ml acetaminophen 120 mg/5 ml alcohol 7.5%
Covangesic, tablet	phenylpropanolamine hydrochloride 12.5 mg phenylephrine hydrochloride 7.5 mg pyrilamine maleate 12.5 mg chlorpheniramine maleate 2.0 mg acetaminophen 275 mg
D Congest-afed, tablet	pseudoephedrine hydrochloride 30 mg
Decapryn, syrup	doxylamine succinate 6.25 mg/5 ml
Demaxin, syrup	phenylephrine hydrochloride 2.5 mg/5 ml chlorpheniramine maleate 1.0 mg/5 ml alcohol 7.5%
Demaxin, repetabs	phenylephrine hydrochloride 20 mg chlorpheniramine 5 mg
D-Feda, syrup	pseudoephedrine hydrochloride 30 mg/ 5 ml
Dristan, tablet	phenylephrine hydrochloride 5 mg chlorpheniramine maleate 2 mg aspirin 325 mg caffeine 16.2 mg
Dristan, time capsule	phenylephrine hydrochloride 20 mg chlorpheniramine maleate 4 mg

D-Sinus, capsule	phenylpropanolamine hydrochloride 18mg acetaminiphen 325 mg
Duadacin, capsule	phenylephrine hydrochloride 5 mg pyrilamine maleate 12.5 mg chlorpheniramine maleate 1 mg salicylamide 200 mg acetaminophen 120 mg ascorbic acid 50 mg caffeine 30 mg
Emagrin Forte, tablet	phenylephrine hydrochloride 5 mg aspirin salicylamide atropine sulfate 0.06 mg caffeine
Endecon, tablet	phenylpropanolamine hydrochloride 25 mg acetaminophen 325 mg
Euphenex, tablet	phenyltoloxamine citrate 25 mg acetaminophen 300 mg caffeine 15 mg
Extendac, capsule	phenylpropanolamine hydrochloride 50 mg pheniramine maleate 12.5 mg chlorpheniramine maleate 1 mg belladonna alkaloids 0.2 mg
Fedahist, tablet	pseudoephedrine hydrochloride 60 mg chlorpheniramine maleate 4 mg
Fedahist, syrup	pseudoephedrine hydrochloride 30 mg/ 5 ml chlorpheniramine maleate 2 mg/5 ml
Fedrazil, tablet	pseudoephedrine hydrochloride 30 mg chlorcyclizine hydrochloride 25 mg
Fendol, tablet	phenylephrine hydrochloride 10 mg salicylamide acetaminophen caffeine

Ginsopan, tablet

phenylpropanolamine hydrochloride
25 mg
phenylephrine hydrochloride 2.5 mg
pyrilamine maleate 12.5 mg
chlorpheniramine maleate 1 mg

Hista-Compound
No. 5, tablet

phenylephrine hydrochloride 4 mg
chlorpheniramine maleate 2 mg
salicylamide 227.5 mg
phenacetin 162.5 mg
caffeine 32.5 mg

Hot Lemon, tablet

phenylephrine hydrochloride 10 mg
chlorpheniramine maleate 2 mg
acetaminophen 600 mg
ascorbic acid 60 mg

Inhiston, tablet

pheniramine maleate 10 mg

Intensin, tablet

acetaminophen 500 mg
chlorpheniramine maleate 2 mg
pseudoephedrin hydrochloride 30 mg

Kiddisan, chewable
tablet

phenylephrine hydrochloride 1.25 mg
chlorpheniramine maleate 2 mg
salicylamide 80 mg
ascorbic acid 30 mg

Midran
Decongestant, tablet

phenylephrine hydrochloride 5 mg
chlorpheniramine maleate 2 mg
salicylamide 97.5 mg
acetaminophen 32.5 mg
caffeine 32.5 mg

Naldegesic, tablet

pseudoephedrine hydrochloride 15 mg
acetaminophen 325 mg

**Nazac Timed-
Disintegration
Decongestant,
capsule**

phenylpropanolamine hydrochloride
50 mg
pheniramine maleate 12.5 mg
chlorpheniramine maleate 1 mg
belladonna alkaloids 0.16 mg

Neo-Synephrine
Compound, tablet

phenylephrine hydrochloride 5 mg
thenyldiamine hydrochloride 7.5 mg
acetaminophen 150 mg
caffeine 15 mg

Neo-Synephrine, elixir	phenylephrine hydrochloride 5 mg/5 ml alcohol 8%
Novafed, syrup	pseudoephedrine hydrochloride 30 mg/ 5 ml alcohol 7.5%
Novafed A, syrup	pseudoephedrine hydrochloride 30 mg/ 5 ml chlorpheniramine maleate 2 mg/5 ml alcohol 5%
Novahistine Elixir	phenylpropanolamine hydrochloride 18.75 mg/5 ml chlorpheniramine maleate 2 mg/5 ml alcohol 5%
Novahistine, tablet	phenylpropanolamine hydrochloride 18.75 mg chlorpheniramine maleate 2 mg
Ornex, capsule	phenylpropanolamine hydrochloride 18 mg acetaminophen 325 mg
Propadrine, capsule	phenylpropanolamine hydrochloride 25 mg
Pyrroxate, capsule, tablet	methoxyphenamine hydrochloride 25 mg chlorpheniramine maleate 2 mg aspirin 227.5 mg phenacetin 162.5 mg caffeine 32.5 mg
Quartets, capsule	phenylpropanolamine hydrochloride 25 mg chlorpheniramine maleate 2 mg dextromethorphan hydrobromide 15 mg vitamin C 25 mg
Rhinex, tablet	phenylephrine hydrochloride 2.5 mg chlorpheniramine maleate 1.25 mg aspirin 150 mg aluminum hydroxide gel magnesium hydroxide

Rhinidrin, tablet   phenylpropanolamine hydrochloride
25 mg
phenyltoloxamine citrate 25 mg
acetaminophen 150 mg
phenacetin 150 mg

Rhinosyn, syrup   chlorpheniramine maleate 4 mg
pseudoephedrine hydrochloride 60 mg

Scot-tussin, syrup   phenylephrine hydrochloride 25 mg/30 cc
pheniramine maleate 80 mg/30 cc
sodium citrate 500 mg/30 cc
sodium salicylate 500 mg/30 cc
caffeine citrate 150 mg/30 cc

Sinac, tablet   phenylpropanolamine hydrochloride
25 mg
phenyltoloxamino citratc 22 mg
acetaminophen 150 mg
phenacetin 150 mg

Sinacet, tablet   pseudoephedrine hydrochloride 15 mg
acetaminophen 325 mg

Sinarest, tablet   phenylephrine hydrochloride 5 mg
chlorpheniramine maleate 1 mg
acetaminophen 300 mg
caffeine 30 mg

Sine-Aid, tablet   phenylephrine hydrochloride 25 mg
aspirin 325 mg

Sine-Off, tablet   phenylpropanolamine hydrochloride
18.75 mg
chlorpheniramine maleate 2 mg
aspirin 500 mg

Sinulin, tablet   phenylpropanolamine hydrochloride
37.5 mg
chlorpheniramine maleate 2 mg
acetaminophen 325 mg
salicylamide 250 mg
homatropine methylbromide 0.75 mg

Sinurex, tablet	phenylpropanolamine hydrochloride 25 mg chlorpheniramine maleate 0.5 mg methapyrilene fumarate 6.25 mg salicylamide 300 mg
Sinustat, tablet	phenylpropanolamine hydrochloride 25 mg phenyltoloxamine dihydrogen citrate 22 mg acetaminophen 325 mg
Sinutab, tablet	phenylpropanolamine hydrochloride 25 mg phenyltoloxamine citrate 22 mg acetaminophen 325 mg
Sinutab II, tablet	phenylpropanolamine hydrochloride 25 mg acetaminophen 325 mg
Sinutab Extra Strength, tablet	phenylpropanolamine hydrochloride 25 mg phenyltoloxamine citrate 22 mg acetaminophen 500 mg
Soltice Decongestant-Analgesic, tablet	phenylpropanolamine hydrochloride 12.5 mg acetaminophen 325 mg
Spantac, capsule	phenylpropanolamine hydrochloride 50 mg chlorpheniramine maleate 4 mg belladonna alkaloids 0.2 mg
St. Joseph Cold Tablet for Children	phenylpropanolamine hydrochloride 3.125 mg aspirin 81 mg
Sudafed, syrup	pseudoephedrine hydrochloride 30 mg/5 ml
Sudafed, tablet	pseudoephedrine hydrochloride 30 mg

Super Anahist, tablet	phenylpropanolamine hydrochloride 25 mg phenyltoloxamine citrate 6.25 mg thonzylamine hydrochloride 6.25 mg acetaminophen 325 mg aspirin 225 mg phenacetin 97.2 mg caffeine
Timed Cold Capsules	phenylpropanolamine hydrochloride 50 mg chlorpheniramine maleate 1 mg pheniramine maleate 12.5 mg belladonna alkaloids 0.16 mg
Triaminic, syrup	phenylpropanolamine hydrochloride 12.5 mg/5 ml pheniramine maleate 6.25 mg/5 ml pyrilamine maleate 6.25 mg/5 ml
Triaminicin, tablet	phenylpropanolamine hydrochloride 25 mg chlorpheniramine maleate 2 mg aspirin 450 mg caffeine 30 mg
Triaminicin, allergy tablet	phenylpropanolamine hydrochloride 37.5 mg chlorpheniramine maleate 4.0 mg
Triaminicin, chewables	phenylpropanolamine hydrochloride 6.25 mg chlorpheniramine maleate 0.5 mg
Ursinus, tablet	phenylpropanolamine hydrochloride 25 mg pheniramine maleate 12.5 mg pyrilamine maleate 12.5 mg aspirin 300 mg
Valihist, capsule	phenylephrine hydrochloride 10 mg pyrilamine maleate 12.5 mg chlorpheniramine maleate 1 mg acetaminophen caffeine

Vasominic TD, tablet

phenylpropanolamine hydrochloride
50 mg
pheniramine maleate 25 mg
pyrilamine maleate 25 mg

Ventilade, syrup

phenylpropanolamine hydrochloride
75 mg
methapyrilene fumarate 25 mg
pyrilamine maleate 25 mg
pheniramine maleate 25 mg
alcohol 5%

4-Way Cold Tablets

phenylpropanolamine hydrochloride
12.5 mg
chlorpheniramine maleate 2 mg
aspirin 324 mg

Viromed, tablet

aspirin 67 mg
chlorpheniramine maleate 1 mg
pseudoephedrine hydrochloride 15 mg
dextromethorphan hydrobromide 7.5 mg
guaifenesin 50 mg

COUGH LOZENGES

Axon

benzocaine 5 mg
cetylpyridinium chloride 2.5 mg

Cepacol

cetylpyridinium chloride 1:1500
benzyl alcohol 0.3%

Cepacol Troches

benzocaine 10 mg
cetylpyridinium chloride 1:1500

Cherry Chloraseptic

phenol
sodium phenolate

Chloraseptic

phenol
sodium phenolate

Colrex Troches

benzocaine 10 mg
cetylpyridinium chloride 2.5 mg

Conex	benzocaine 5 mg cetylpyridinium chloride 0.5 mg methylparaben 2 mg propylparaben 0.5 mg
Creozets	beechwood creosote white pine ipecac menthol cascara wild cherry alcohol 1%
Hold	benzocaine dextromethorphan hydrobromide
Listerine	hexylresorcinol 2.4 mg eucalyptol menthol
Listerine Cough Control	benzocaine 2.5 mg dextromethorphan hydrobromide 7.5 mg
Meloids Pastilles	licorice 98 mg sugar 48 mg capsicum 2 mg menthol 1.8 mg
Oracin	benzocaine 6.25 mg menthol 0.10% sorbitol base
Oradex-C	benzocaine 10 mg cetylpyridinium chloride 2.5 mg
Robitussin-DM Cough Calmers	dextromethorphan hydrobromide 7.5 mg guaifenesin 50 mg
Romilar Cough Discs	dextromethorphan hydrobromide 5 mg benzyl alcohol 0.5%
Semets	benzocaine 3 mg cetylpyridinium chloride 1:1500
Sepo	benzocaine

Silence is Golden	dextromethorphan hydrobromide 5 mg
Spec-T Sore Throat Anesthetic	benzocaine 10 mg
Spec-T Sore Throat/ Cough Suppressant	benzocaine 10 mg dextromethorphan hydrobromide 10 mg
Spec-T Sore Throat/ Decongestant	benzocaine 10 mg phenylephrine hydrochloride 5 mg phenylpropanolamine hydrochloride 10.5 mg
Spongiacaine	benzocaine
Sucrets	hexylresorcinol 2.4 mg
Synthaloids	benzocaine calcium-iodine complex
Teeds	benzocaine 10 mg chlorophyll
Thantis	meralein sodium 8.1 mg salicyl alcohol 64.8 mg
Thriocaine, lozenge	benzocaine 5 mg cetylpyridinium chloride 0.5 mg
Throat Discs	capsicum peppermint anise cubeb glycyrrhiza extract linseed
Trocaine	benzocaine 5 mg
Trokettes	benzocaine 10 mg cetylpyridinium chloride 1:3000 cetalkonium chloride 1:3000
Vicks Cough Silencers	benzocaine 1 mg dextromethorphan hydrobromide 2.5 mg/ drop menthol

	anethole
	peppermint oil
Vicks Formula 44 Cough Discs	benzocaine 1.25 mg
	dextromethorphan hydrobromide 5 mg
	menthol
	anethole
	peppermint oil
Vicks Medi-trating	benzocaine 5 mg
	cetylpyridinium chloride 1.66 mg
	menthol
	camphor
	eucalyptus oil

8. Conjunctivitis
(Red, irritated eyes)

What is conjunctivitis?
The eye is truly a miraculous part of the body, a super lens that constantly relays images to the brain. It has several functions and a variety of parts.

One specific part is the conjunctiva, a fine layer of tissue that lines the inside of the eyelids and the front of the eye. Thin, delicate, and loaded with tiny blood vessels, the conjunctiva is essentially invisible when normal. But, when irritated, the blood vessels enlarge and get prominently red; and the eyelids become puffy, itchy and uncomfortable. The reddening, swelling, and itching are all components of conjunctivitis, an inflammation of the conjunctiva of the eye and eyelids.

What causes conjunctivitis?
The most common causes of conjunctivitis are chemical irritants, like smoke, and other forms of pollution that fill the air, invade the eye, and pester the conjunctiva. Pollen and other airborne allergens (see Chapter 3) will also adversely affect the eye, producing a specific form of conjunctivitis called allergic conjunctivitis. Bacterial conjunctivitis, as the name implies, is caused by bacteria which infect the surface of the eye to produce pus and a crusting discharge, in addition to the redness and swelling that are common to allergic and chemical conjunctivitis. And, the eye irritation that frequently accompanies flus and colds is usually caused by the invading virus and is consequently named viral conjunctivitis.

102

Thus, the causes of conjunctivitis include chemical irritants, pollen, bacteria, and viruses, all of which produce the common symptoms of redness, swelling, itching, and pain, plus purulent discharges in the case of bacterial involvement.

What should be done for conjunctivitis?
Treatment depends on the variety of the conjunctivitis. Bacterial forms require antibiotic therapy and the evaluation of a physician. In these cases, the presence of pus, moderate to severe redness, and crusty stickiness of the eyelids should prompt medical investigation. For the conjunctival irritation associated with colds and flus, oral decongestants, that are taken to relieve stuffy nose and sinuses, will also help to reduce the eye irritation. Finally, for mild cases of chemical or allergic conjunctivitis, eye drops will help.

What eye medications will relieve simple conjunctivitis?
There are four primary medications for simple conjunctivitis.
Ephedrine: Ephedrine is a vasoconstrictor drug that decongests or reduces the enlarged prominent blood vessels of the conjunctivita. The action of ephedrine is short lived when compared to other eye decongestants. It also produces a "rebound effect," which manifests itself as a secondary enlargement of the blood vessels after the first effects of the ephedrine have worn off.
Phenylephrine: This drug, which is closely related to ephedrine, has a longer duration of action and has been used successfully to relieve vascular congestion of the eyes. Its one major drawback is the tendency to break down when exposed to air. Thus, prolonged storage of this drug will greatly reduce its effectiveness.
Naphazoline: Naphazoline is a long-acting ocular decongestant, but concentrations found in most OTC eye products are small and tend to be ineffective.
Tetrahydrozoline: Similar to naphazoline in its chemical

composition, tetrahydrozoline is also long acting and very effective when used in the proper concentrations. Rebound symptoms do not occur, and the drug is more stable than phenylephrine.

RECOMMENDED TREATMENT
Tetrahydrozoline in a concentration equal to 0.05 percent provides an excellent means of reducing the congestion and irritation of mild uncomplicated conjunctivitis.

COMMENTS AND CAUTIONS
Anyone suffering from glaucoma should consult a doctor before using an eye decongestant. Following the use of these products, an acute attack of narrow angle glaucoma may occur and cause permanent damage to the eye.

EYE DECONGESTANTS
Boldface: Recommended

Allerest	naphazoline hydrochloride 0.012% thimerosal 0.005% boric acid sodium carbonate potassium chloride camphor zinc sulfate
Clear Eyes	naphazoline hydrochloride 0.012% methylcellulose edetate disodium 0.1% benzalkonium chloride 0.01% boric acid sodium borate
Collyrium Drops	ephedrine sulfate 0.1% thimerosal 0.002% boric acid sodium borate antipyrine 0.4% sodium salicylate 0.056%

Degest	phenylephrine hydrochloride 0.2% edetate disodium 0.05% benzalkonium chloride 0.01%
Eye Cool	phenylephrine hydrochloride 0.08% edetate disodium 0.05% thimerosal 0.002% sodium borate boric acid menthol eucalyptus oil sodium chloride sodium bisulfite
Eye Gene	phenylephrine hydrochloride boric acid sodium borate sodium chloride sodium bisulfite camphor peppermint water thimerosal benzalkonium chloride
Eye Genic Spray	phenylephrine hydrochloride boric acid sodium borate sodium chloride sodium bisulfite camphor peppermint water thimerosal benzalkonium chloride
20/20 Eye Drops	naphazoline hydrochloride 0.012% thimerosal 0.005% boric acid sodium carbonate potassium chloride zinc sulfate
Isopto-Frin	phenylephrine hydrochloride 0.12% hydroxypropyl methylcellulose 0.5% benzethonium chloride sodium citrate sodium phosphate sodium biphosphate

Murine 2

tetrahydrazoline hydrochloride 0.05%
boric acid
methylcellulose
sodium acetate
disodium edetate 0.1%
benzalkonium chloride 0.01%

Murine

benzalkonium chloride 0.004%
thimerosal 0.001%
potassium borate
potassium bicarbonate
hydrastine
berberine
glycerin

Naphcon

naphazoline hydrochloride 0.012%
benzalkonium chloride 0.01%

Ocusol Drops

phenylephrine hydrochloride
methylcellulose
benzalkonium chloride
boric acid
sodium borate
sodium chloride

Phenylzin

phenylephrine hydrochloride 0.012%
hydroxypropyl methylcellulose 0.1%
benzalkonium chloride 0.01%
edetate disodium 0.01%
boric acid 1.1%
sodium carbonate 0.02%
zinc sulfate 0.25%
sodium bisulfite 0.01%
potassium chloride

Prefrin

phenylephrine hydrochloride 0.12%
polyvinyl alcohol 1.4%
benzalkonium chloride 0.004%
sodium phosphate
sodium biphosphate
antipyrine 0.1%

Prefrin Z	phenylephrine hydrochloride 0.12% polyvinyl alcohol 1.4% thimerosal 0.005% sodium hydroxide sodium citrate zinc sulfate 0.25% sodium chloride sodium bisulfite
Tear-efrin	phenylephrine hydrochloride 0.1% hydroxypropyl methylcellulose 0.5% benzalkonium chloride 0.01% edetate disodium 0.01% sodium bisulfite 0.05% sodium chloride
Visine	tetrahydrozoline hydrochloride 0.05% edetate disodium 0.1% benzalkonium chloride 0.01% boric acid sodium borate sodium chloride
Zincfrin	phenylephrine hydrochloride 0.12% benzalkonium chloride 0.01% barbital barbital sodium zinc sulfate 0.25%

9. Constipation

What is constipation?

Constipation, a very common and particularly annoying ailment, is the inability to move the bowels when the need to defecate is present. However, because of the great variation in normal bowel habits, a clarification of the problem is necessary.

For example, just because a person doesn't have a bowel movement for three days does not mean that person is constipated. In fact, many perfectly normal people have only one bowel movement every three days because that's all they need; that's their normal pattern. Other people have one bowel movement everyday, while still others might have three a day. Each is normal.

Therefore, constipation is real only when the regular pattern is upset and the ability to defecate does not accompany the need.

Under normal circumstances what causes a bowel movement?

A bowel movement occurs when digestive waste material accumulates in the rectum, the last part of the large intestine. Normally, when this happens, the rectum responds with forceful contractions that push the waste out of the body. The same contractions result following a meal, especially breakfast, when food entering the stomach triggers a nerve reflex that stimulates the rectum to evacuate. Coffee, a particularly strong irritant, also has this stimulatory effect on many people in the morning.

What causes constipation, the inability to move the bowels?

As with most medical problems, there are several causes of constipation. Here are eight of the most common.

Diets: Simple constipation may result from the inadequate consumption of "bulky" foods, that is, foods which leave considerable residue in the intestines following digestion. Lettuce, spinach, cabbage, and other high-fiber vegetables are all examples of bulky foods. Furthermore, foods such as cheese, which tend to harden the stools and promote difficult bowel movements, occasionally cause constipation if eaten in excess.

Emotions: Interestingly, one of the most common causes of diarrhea is also a frequent cause of constipation. Spastic colitis, an illness associated with emotional and psychological stress, can lead to either diarrhea or constipation, because stimulation of the rectum is irregular and so are the rectal contractions that lead to a bowel movement. Consequently, food and waste material within the bowel are not propelled forward at the normal rate. They either move too quickly, producing diarrhea, or to slowly, resulting in constipation.

Inactive bowels: Inactive bowels is a problem that arises when the large intestine loses the muscular strength it once had. Being weaker, it cannot hold its normal shape or contract forcefully enough to adequately move waste materials. Bowel movements are reduced and waste simply collects in the intestines. Bedridden individuals and inactive people suffer from this condition.

Desensitization: When the natural urge to defecate is suppressed because of hectic schedules, unavailable bathroom facilities, and the like, the bowel loses its sensitivity, and the normal mechanisms that promote active bowel movements are also lost. Although everyone faces this problem occasionally, those people who regularly suppress the normal urge will frequently suffer from constipation.

Medicines: Numerous drugs that are taken daily can either disrupt normal intestinal contractions or harden the stools; two actions that often lead to constipation. For example, aluminum hydroxide and calcium carbonate, substances found in a multitude of antacid preparations, tend to harden the stools, making them difficult to pass. Opium and the anticholinergic drugs, which are frequently found in the antidiarrheal products, slow down the normal intestinal pulsations and occasionally promote decreased bowel movements. Constipation is the result in both cases.

Post-diarrhea: Following a bout of diarrhea, several days may pass before a regular bowel movement occurs. There are two major reasons for this change. First, during the diarrhea attack, the bowel completely empties, and a few days are needed for waste material to accumulate again. Secondly, as described above, the medications that are taken to control diarrhea may reduce bowel movements enough to cause constipation.

Quitting cigarettes: Just as food in the stomach or accumulated waste in the rectum activates bowel contractions that lead to bowel movements, smoking may accomplish the same goal. This is why smokers often experience the need to move their bowels after smoking a cigarette, especially that first cigarette in the morning. Thus, when a person quits smoking, the stimulant effect that tobacco has had on the bowel is removed, and constipation may occur until the intestinal tract finds a replacement stimulus.

Physical diseases: The reasons for constipation described above are common and relatively insignificant when compared with some of the physical problems that may affect the intestines, causing decreased bowel movements. Irritation of the anus or sensitive hemorrhoids may foster constipation, because bowel movements become painful and, consequently, are avoided as much as possible. Intestinal obstruction or blockage—which occurs with hard feces impacted in the rectum or with twisted segments of bowel, as well as with tumors and a variety of other causes—will also produce constipation, because waste material simply cannot move past the point of interference.

Other disease processes in the abdomen, gallbladder problems, appendicitis, infections of the ovaries, and diverticulitis, just to name a few, may also lead to a reduction in bowel movements. Finally, physical problems in the nervous system that prevent the nerve stimulation required for normal bowel movements will also give rise to constipation.

Are there other symptoms that are commonly associated with constipation?

Yes there are. Simple constipation may be accompanied by mild cramps, pain, or tenderness. In more extreme cases when the large intestine is greatly distended with waste, bloating may be experienced along with headaches, loss of appetite, and fatigue.

If a serious physical illness, such as a large bowel cancer with obstruction, is causing the constipation, symptoms will probably be more complicated and severe and they are likely to be present before the constipation. These symptoms include nausea, vomiting, weight loss, bleeding from the rectum, fever, and persistent pain.

Can the proper diet reduce the possibility of constipation?

Absolutely! Constipation, diverticulosis, and cancer of the colon are much more common in people who eat foods that are low in fiber content. High fiber, bulky foods, such as vegetables, grains, fruits and nuts, add large quantities of residue to intestinal waste and promote good strong intestinal contractions and normal natural bowel movements.

In the United States, where meat and potatoes often replace grains and vegetables, diets tend to be low in fiber content. Intestinal problems are therefore quite common, and that may help to explain why cancer of the colon has become one of the major killers of Americans. People who suffer from occasional constipation but have no known physical diseases of the bowel can develop more consistent bowel habits by eating bulkier foods and, at the same time, reduce their chances of developing serious bowel diseases, such as cancer.

How can bulky foods prevent cancer?

Small sites of cancer develop in the body constantly. Usually, they are quickly suppressed by our natural defense mechanisms and never have a chance to grow into the large tumors that take lives. It is thought that small concentrations of cancer cells also develop in the intestines, but that normally they are either sloughed off as new cells replace old cells or scraped away by bulky food residues as they pass through the bowel. Therefore, people who consume high fiber foods are less likely to develop intestinal cancer.

Can exercise improve bowel habits?
Absolutely! Exercise is a primary need for normal body functions. By toning muscles, especially those of the abdomen, the intestines will also become stronger and will perform their functions more efficiently. In fact, the lack of daily exercise frequently leads to constipation.

Can laxatives aid bowel movements?
Laxatives are acceptable aids which can be taken to promote bowel movements if they are used with discretion. For occasional irregularity that is not associated with serious underlying physical problems, laxatives will promote emptying of the bowel and relief of the minor discomforts of constipation. It cannot be overemphasized, however, that laxatives should only be used to overcome occasional constipation. They should not be used to promote daily bowel movements.

There seem to be many laxatives available over the counter. Is one just about the same as another?
Absolutely not. The ingredients of different laxatives vary considerably. Here are the seven major forms of laxative treatments and the medications they encompass.

Bulk formers: Bulk formers are laxatives that exert an effect by producing expansion of the stomach and bowel. Once swallowed, these substances balloon to many times their original size, distending the stomach much as a large meal will. They consist primarily of carboxymethylcellulose, methylcellulose, polycarbophil, and psyllium.

The bulk producers must be consumed with a large glass of water to prevent blockage of the intestines. Because of this possibility of intestinal obstruction, these agents should not be used by people who have intestinal narrowing, abdominal adhesions, or swallowing difficulties.

Emollients: Emollients work by softening fecal material with the water and fat normally present in the intestines. Dioctyl sodium sulfosuccinate, dioctyl calcium sulfosuccinate, and poloxamer-188 are the common emollient medications available over the counter. Their use is intended to prevent, rather than relieve, constipation in older individuals who generally form hard, dry stools and have difficulty passing them.

Enemas: Tap water and saltwater enemas produce their laxative effect by filling the large intestine with fluid, thereby stretching the intestinal walls and stimulating the nerve reflexes that promote bowel movements. Soapy enemas will produce the above effect, but, in addition, irritate the bowel walls and stimulate reflex rectal contractions. Oil enemas lubricate and soften fecal waste, thus aiding their passage. When used properly, enemas are a very effective and relatively natural way to cleanse and empty the bowel.

Lubricants: Lubricant laxatives include mineral and plant oils that are taken orally. These substances prevent the absorption of water from intestinal waste, and thus prevent dry, hard stools and the subsequent accompanying constipation. With continued use, however, mineral oil may be significantly absorbed from the gut and is capable of producing abnormal changes in the liver, spleen, and lymph glands. Furthermore, it has been shown that chronic mineral-oil ingestion prevents the natural absorption of calcium, phosphate, vitamin A, and vitamin D from the intestines.

Saline laxatives: Saline laxatives are composed of magnesium and phosphate compounds that are taken orally and become intermixed with intestinal waste material. They tend to hold water within the intestines and, in this way, stimulate bowel movements. Unfortunately, magnesium is partially absorbed from the intestines and must be removed from the body by the kidneys. Since people with kidney disease might not be able to effectively eliminate absorbed magnesium, they should not use the saline laxatives that contain this compound. The phosphate laxatives that contain high sodium concentrations, should not be used by people on salt-free diets.

Stimulants: By irritating the intestinal lining and stimulating nerve reflexes, stimulant laxatives cause increased rectal contractions and bowel movements. The members of this group of laxatives are aloe, bisacodyl, cascara, castor oil, danthron, phenolphthalein, and senna. The use of aloe is not recommended because this substance is too irritating.

Bisacodyl selectively acts on the lining of the large bowel and stimulates the nerves located there. Since this substance is not absorbed from the intestines, it exerts no generalized effect on the body. Both suppository and oral forms are available over the counter.

Cascara and senna are two common stimulant laxatives that are widely used today. Unfortunately, they are absorbed from the intestines and must subsequently be removed from the body in some way. Senna can be found in the milk of nursing mothers and occasionally produces diarrhea in their breast-fed infants.

Castor oil produces an irritation of the small intestine, which causes increased pulsations of that part of the bowel and subsequent defecation. The use of this oil is discouraged because it promotes excessive loss of nutritionally valuable solids and liquids by rushing foods through the small intestine too quickly for adequate digestion and absorption.

Danthron, like bisacodyl, produces its laxative effect by a direct action on the lining of the large bowel. Unlike bisacodyl, it is absorbed in the small bowel, metabolized in the liver, and excreted by the kidneys.

Phenolphthalein causes increased bowel contractions of both the large and small intestines which lead to defecation. A portion of this substance is absorbed from the intestines and excreted in the urine, at times imparting a pink or red color to that fluid. Several toxic conditions may result from the use of phenolphthalein compounds, however. Occasionally excessive bowel movements and diarrhea will result, leading to dangerous fluid and electrolyte (potassium and sodium) loss. Allergic reactions have also been encountered and range from mild skin rashes to serious heart and lung problems. Osteomalacia, a bone disorder, has occurred with excessive use of phenolphthalein laxatives, but this condition has corrected itself when the laxative was discontinued.

Suppositories: Laxative suppositories contain bisacodyl, dioctyl sodium sulfosuccinate, glycerin, senna, and carbon dioxide releasing substances. These ingredients act in different ways to induce bowel movements, but the method of administration is basically the same. The suppository is inserted into the rectum and, as it melts, it releases its specific laxative ingredient.

Glycerin suppositories have been used successfully for years and usually stimulate bowel movements within an hour. Carbon dioxide suppositories are relatively new. Working much like an enema, they promote bowel movements by filling the colon with harmless carbon dioxide gas instead of water or oils.

RECOMMENDED TREATMENT

In view of the great variety of OTC laxatives available, the proper choice depends on the individual and the specific problem. When dry, hard stools are the cause of constipation, or when hemorrhoids and anal irritation make bowel movements painful, a stool softener such as dioctyl sodium sulfosuccinate or bulk producers are wisely used. By softening fecal material, less pain is generated as the stool passes over sensitive hemorrhoids or anal sores. Secondary constipation is then avoided.

Most other cases of constipation are best treated by suppositories or enemas. Personally, I prefer suppositories because of their easy administration and lack of messy complications. Glycerin, bisacodyl, and carbon dioxide forms are safe and effective.

COMMENTS AND CAUTIONS

As I mentioned previously, constipation may be associated with serious physical disease of the bowel, in which case it should be treated by a physician as soon as possible. Laxatives should not be used in these cases because they may instigate additional complications. A simple rule to remember: When constipation is associated with severe abdominal pains, fever, nausea, vomiting, weight loss, or thin, pencil-like stools, laxatives should be avoided, and a doctor should be consulted.

LAXATIVE MEDICATIONS
Boldface: Recommended

Afko-Lube, capsule	dioctyl sodium sulfosuccinate 100 mg
Afko-Lube Lax, capsule	dioctyl sodium sulfosuccinate 100 mg casanthranol 30 mg
Agoral, emulsion	phenolphthalein 1.3 mg/100 mg mineral oil agar gel tragacanth acacia
Alophen, tablet	phenolphthalein 60 mg
Amlax, tablet	phenolphthalein 32.5 mg cascara sagrada extract 32.5 mg bile salts 65 mg
Black Draught, tablet, syrup, granules	senna 300 mg/tablet senna 175 mg/1 ml senna 660 mg/1 g
Caroid and Bile Salts with Phenolphthalein, tablet	phenolphthalein 32.4 mg cascara sagrada extract 48.6 mg bile salts 70 mg papaya extract 75 mg capsicum 6.5 mg
Carter's Little Pills, tablet	aloe 16 mg podophyllum 4 mg
Casakol, capsule	poloxamer-188 250 mg casanthranol 30 mg
Casa-Laud, tablet	dioctyl sodium sulfosuccinate 100 mg casanthranol 30 mg

Cas-Evac, liquid	cascara sagrada 200 mg/100 ml alcohol 18%
Casyllium, powder	cascara fluid extract 15 ml/30 g psyllium husk 20.5 g/30 g prune powder 6 g/30 g
Ceo-Two, suppository	sodium bicarbonate potassium bitartrate polyethylene glycol
Colace, capsule, liquid, syrup	dioctyl sodium sulfosuccinate 50–100 mg dioctyl sodium sulfosuccinate 1% dioctyl sodium sulfosuccinate 20 mg/5 ml
Coloctyl, capsule	dioctyl sodium sulfosuccinate 100 mg
Comfolax, capsule	dioctyl sodium sulfosuccinate 100 mg
Comfolax Plus, capsule	dioctyl sodium sulfosuccinate 100 mg casanthranol 30 mg
Constiban, capsule	dioctyl sodium sulfosuccinate 100 mg casanthranol 30 mg
Correctol, tablet	dioctyl sodium sulfoscuccinate 100 mg yellow phenolphthalein 64.8 mg
Decholin, tablet	dehydrocholic acid 250 mg
Dialose, capsule	dioctyl sodium sulfosuccinate 100 mg carboxymethylcellulose sodium 400 mg
Dialose Plus, capsule	dioctyl sodium sulfosuccinate 100 mg carboxymethylcellulose sodium 400 mg casanthranol 30 mg
Dilox	dioctyl sodium sulfosuccinate 250 mg
Diomedicone, tablet	dioctyl sodium sulfosuccinate 50 mg
Dio-Sul, capsule	dioctyl sodium sulfosuccinate 100 mg
Diothron, capsule	dioctyl sodium sulfosuccinate 100 mg casanthranol 30 mg

Disanthrol, capsule	dioctyl sodium sulfosuccinate 100 mg casanthranol 30 mg
Disolan, capsule	dioctyl sodium sulfosuccinate 100 mg casanthranol 30 mg
Disolan Forte, capsule	dioctyl sodium sulfosuccinate 100 mg carboxymethylcellulose sodium 400 mg casanthranol 30 mg
Disonate, capsule	dioctyl sodium sulfosuccinate 60, 100, 240 mg
liquid	dioctyl sodium sulfosuccinate 10 mg/1 ml
syrup	dioctyl sodium sulfosuccinate 20 mg/5 ml
Disoplex, capsule	dioctyl sodium sulfosuccinate 100 mg carboxymethylcellulose sodium 400 mg
Doctate, capsule	dioctyl sodium sulfosuccinate 100, 300 mg
Doctate-P, capsule	dioctyl sodium sulfosuccinate 60 mg danthron 40 mg
Dorbane, tablet	danthron 75 mg
Dorbantyl, capsule	dioctyl sodium sulfosuccinate 50 mg danthron 25 mg
Dorbantyl Forte, capsule	dioctyl sodium sulfosuccinate 100 mg danthron 50 mg
Doxan, tablet	dioctyl sodium sulfosuccinate 60 mg danthron 50 mg
Doxidan, capsule	dioctyl calcium sulfosuccinate 60 mg danthron 50 mg
Doxinate, capsule	dioctyl sodium sulfosuccinate 60, 240 mg
Dr. Caldwell's Senna Laxative, liquid	senna 412 mg/5 ml peppermint oil 0.95 mg/5 ml alcohol 4.5%
Dual Formula Feen- A-Mint, tablet	dioctyl sodium sulfosuccinate 100 mg yellow phenolphthalein 64.8 mg

Dulcolax, tablet	bisacodyl 5 mg
Dulcolax, suppository	bisacodyl 10 mg
Effersyllium, powder	psyllium hydrocolloid 3 g/7 g
Enemeez, enema	sodium biphosphate 16 g/100 ml sodium phosphate 6 g/100 ml methylparaben 100 mg/100 ml propylparaben 100 mg/100 ml
Espotabs, tablet	yellow phenolphthalein
Evac-Q-Mag, liquid	magnesium citrate 300 ml
Evac-Q-Sert, suppository	carbon-dioxide releasing
Evac-Q-Tabs, tablet	phenolphthalein 130 mg
Evac-U-Gen, tablet	yellow phenolphthalein 97.2 mg
Ex-Lax, chocolate tablet	yellow phenolphthalein 97.2 mg
Feen-A-Mint, mint	yellow phenolphthalein 97.2 mg
chewable tablet	yellow phenolphthalein 97.2 mg
chewing gum	yellow phenolphthalein 75 mg
pills	dioctyl sodium sulfosuccinate 100 mg yellow phenophthalein 65 mg
Fleet Bagenema	liquid castile soap 19.7 ml
Fleet Enema	sodium biphosphate 19 g/118 ml sodium phosphate 7 g/118 ml
Fleet Enema Oil Retention	mineral oil 118 ml
Fleet Pediatric, enema	sodium biphosphate 9.5 g/59 ml sodium phosphate 3.5 g/59 ml
Fletcher's Castoria, liquid	senna 6.5%

Gardalax, capsule	dioctyl sodium sulfosuccinate 100 mg casanthranol 30 mg
Gentlax, tablet	senna concentrate 326 mg guar gum 1 g polygalacturonic acid 100 mg
Gentlax, granules	senna concentrates 326 mg/tsp guar gum 1 g/tsp polygalacturonic acid 100 mg/tsp
Gentlax B, tablet	senna concentrate 108.7 mg guar gum 333 mg
Gentlax B, granules	senna concentrate 326.1 mg/tsp guar gum 1 g/tsp
Gentlax S, tablet	dioctyl sodium sulfosuccinate 50 mg senna concentrate 187 mg
Glysennid, tablet	sennosides A and B 12 mg
G-W Emulsoil, instant mix	castor oil 30 ml
G-W Emulsoil, liquid	castor oil 60 ml
Haley's M-O, emulsion	magnesium hydroxide 75% mineral oil 25%
Hydrocil, powder	psyllium 40% karaya gum 10% dextrose 50%
Hydrocil Fortified, powder	casanthranol 60 mg/6 g psyllium 40% karaya gum 10% dextrose 50%
Hydrolose, syrup	methylcellulose 591 g/30 ml
Imbicoll, granules	cascara sagrada 1.27 ml/ 7 g karaya gum 86%
Kondremul, microemulsion	mineral oil 55% chondrus

Konsyl, powder	blond psyllium 100%
L.A., formula	blond psyllium 50%
Laxadan, tablet	dioctyl sodium sulfosuccinate 100 mg bisacodyl 5 mg
Laxadan, suppository	bisacodyl 10 mg
Laxative H, capsule	dioctyl sodium sulfosuccinate 100 mg casanthranol 30 mg
Laxsil, suspension	magnesium hydroxide 1.25 g/15 ml simethicone 100 mg/15 ml
Liqui-Doss, liquid	dioctyl sodium sulfosuccinate 60 mg/15 cc mineral oil
Magcyl, capsule	dioctyl sodium sulfosuccinate 100 mg danthron 25 mg
Maltsupex	malt soup extract 750 mg
Metamucil, Instant Mix, powder packets	psyllium mucilloid 3.7 g citric acid sodium bicarbonate (250 mg sodium)
Metamucil, powder	psyllium mucilloid 50% dextrose 50%
Milkinol, liquid	dioctyl sodium sulfosuccinate 3.3 mg/5 ml mineral oil 4.75 ml/ 5 ml
Modane, tablet, liquid	danthron 75 mg danthron 10 ml
Modane Mild, tablet	danthron 37.5 mg
Mucilose, granules, flakes	psyllium 50% dextrose 50%
Nature's Remedy Juniors, tablet	cascara sagrada 42 mg aloe 48 mg

Nature's Remedy Regular and Candy Coated, tablets	cascara sagrada 127 mg aloe 143 mg
Neo-Cultol, suspension	mineral oil jelly
Neoloid, emulsion	castor oil 36.4 mg
Nujol, liquid	mineral oil
Oxathalein, tablet	phenolphthalein 32 mg cascara sagrada extract 32 mg aloin 8 mg
Peri-Colace, capsule	dioctyl sodium sulfosuccinate 100 mg casanthranol 30 mg
Peri-Colace, syrup	dioctyl sodium sulfosuccinate 20 mg/5 ml casanthranol 10 mg/5 ml
Peristim Forte, capsule	casanthranol 90 mg
Petrogalar, liquid	mineral oil 65%
Petrogalar cascara, liquid	cascara sagrada 13.2% mineral oil 65%
Petrogalar, emulsion	cascara 13.2% mineral oil 65% agar sodium alginate acacia glycerin
Petrogalar, emulsion (phenolphthalein)	phenolphthalein 0.3% mineral oil 65% agar sodium alginate acacia glycerin
Petrogalar, liquid (phenolphthalein)	phenolphthalein 0.3% mineral oil 65%

Petro-Syllium No. 1 Plain, liquid	psyllium husk 750 mg/100 g mineral oil 47.5 mg/100 g
Petro-Syllium No. 2, with phenolphthalein, liquid	phenolphthalein 243.8 mg/30 ml psyllium husk mineral oil
Phenolax Wafer, tablet	phenolphthalein 243.8 mg/30 ml
Phillips Milk of Magnesia, suspension	magnesium hydroxide 2.27–2.62 g/30 ml peppermint oil 1.166 mg/30 ml
Phillips Milk of Magnesia, tablet	magnesium hydroxide 311 mg peppermint oil 1.166 mg
Phospho-Soda, liquid	sodium biphosphate 48 g/100 ml sodium phosphate 18 g/100 ml sweeteners and flavors
Plova (plain), powder	psyllium 100%
Plova (flavored), powder	psyllium 50% dextrose 50%
Polykol, capsule	poloxamer-188 25 mg
Prulet, tablet	white phenolphthalein 60 mg or 30 mg
Rectalac, enema	dioctyl potassium sulfosuccinate 5% glycerin 76% soft soap 5%
Regul-Aid, capsule	dioctyl sodium sulfosuccinate 100 mg
Regul-Aid, syrup	dioctyl sodium sulfosuccinate 20 mg/5 ml
Regutol, tablet	dioctyl sodium sulfosuccinate 100 mg
Sal Hepatica, granules	monosodium phosphate
Saraka, granules	stereulia frangula

Senokap DSS, capsule	dioctyl sodium sulfosuccinate 50 mg senna concentrate 163 mg
Senokot, granules	senna concentrate 326 mg/tsp
Senokot, suppository	senna concentrate 652 mg
Senokot, syrup	senna concentrate 218 mg/5 ml
Senokot, tablet	senna concentrate 187 mg
Senokot-S, tablet	dioctyl sodium sulfosuccinate 50 mg senna concentrate 187 mg
Senokot with Psyllium, powder	senna concentrate 326 mg/5 ml psyllium 1 g/5 ml
Serutan, powder	vegetable hemicellulose from plantago
Serutan, granules	vegetable hemicellulose from plantago
Siblin, granules	psyllium husks 62.4% sugar caramel sodium chloride
S-K Bisacodyl	bisacodyl 5 mg
Squibb glycerin, suppositories	glycerin
Stimulax, capsule	dioctyl sodium sulfosuccinate 250 mg cascara 30 mg
Surfak, capsule	dioctyl calcium sulfosuccinate 50–240 mg
Swiss Kriss, powder	senna herbs
Syllact, powder	psyllium husks 50% dextrose 50%
Syllamalt, powder	psyllium husks 50% malt soup extract 50%

Syllamalt Effervescent, powder	psyllium husks 25% malt soup extract 25% dextrose sodium bicarbonate citric acid
Theralax, suppository	bisacodyl 10 mg triglyceride base
Therlax, tablet	bisacodyl 5 mg
Tonelax, tablet	danthron 75 mg calcium pantothenate 25 mg
Tucks Saf-Tip Oil Retention Enema	mineral oil
Tucks Saf-Tip Phosphate Enema	sodium biphosphate 16 g/100 ml sodium phosphate 6 g/100 ml
Vacuetts Adult, suppository	sodium biphosphate sodium acid pyrophosphate sodium bicarbonate polyethylene glycols
Wyeth Bisacodyl, suppository	bisacodyl 10 mg
X-Prep, liquid	senna extract
X-Prep, powder	senna concentrate

10. Contact Dermatitis
(Poison Ivy and Poison Oak)

What is contact dermatitis?
Contact dermatitis, or allergic dermatitis, is an inflammation of the skin that results from contact with certain naturally occurring and synthetic substances, that doctors call sensitizers or allergens.

What substances act as sensitizers and cause contact dermatitis?
Just about any substance can cause contact dermatitis. However, there are several agents that prompt allergic responses quite regularly: poison oak and poison ivy are prime examples. Other members of the plant family that are frequently incriminated include poison sumac, primrose, ragweed, chrysanthemum, teak, mahogany, kapok, Japanese lacquer tree (including the lacquer made from the tree and used on household furniture), and the cashew nut tree. Among the fruits and vegetables, we find citrus fruits and mangos producing dermatitis on certain individuals.

Chemical substances will also cause allergic skin lesions. The most frequent culprits are metal compounds composed of mercury, nickel, and chromium.

Cosmetics play a distinct role, too, manifested by the allergic response that occasionally occurs following the use of hair sprays, hair dyes, perfumes, deodorants, and antiperspirants.

Household products (cleansers, oils, waxes, and polishes) and clothing made from wool, silk, leather, fur, or synthetic fibers sensitize also.

126

In what way do these substances produce an allergic skin response?
An allergic reaction of the skin begins when allergens combine with specific skin proteins and set in motion a complex sequence of events intended to neutralize the invading foreign substance. When the antigen is discovered by white blood cells, combatting or neutralizing antibodies are produced. The antibodies then attach themselves to the antigen (antibody-antigen complexes are the result of the combination) and, in so doing, inactivate the originally toxic sensitizer. However, some individuals react inappropriately. The antibody-antigen complex chemically causes the excessive release of inflammatory substances like histamines that act on blood vessels, causing them to swell and leak fluid.

Some people will develop skin allergies while other will not. Why?
The people who develop contact allergic dermatitis must first be exposed to an appropriate sensitizer, then have the exact protein fractions in the skin and develop the necessary complete antigen (sensitizer plus protein). Finally they must activate antibody production and exhibit faulty antibody responses. If any one of these conditions is not met, contact dermatitis does not arise. Therefore, those people who never come in contact with an appropriate sensitizer or fail to form a complete antigen will never suffer from contact dermatitis. Furthermore, if no antibodies are produced or if the antibodies that are manufactured by white blood cells neutralize the sensitizer inadequately, contact dermatitis is avoided. Thus, a variety of factors participates in the development of contact dermatitis, and it is the individual constitution of each person that determines whether all of these factors are present.

What are the signs and symptoms of contact dermatitis?
Following exposure to a sensitizer, redness and swelling will occur in about twenty-four hours. Very small (1/32 inch) to

very large (1 inch) water blisters may then form, pop, and crust over with a fluid discharge that dries and hardens. Itching is usually pronounced.

The most common sites are the exposed areas of the body, the face, neck, arms, legs, hands, and feet—although any part of the body where skin and sensitizer meet is open territory. Frequently, the site will provide an important clue as to the identity of the offending substance. For example, if both feet develop the characteristics of contact dermatitis consider the socks, shoes, or any substances applied to the feet as a possible cause. If the face, hands, and upper chest are involved, chances are good that the responsible agent is a plant or chemical. When the trunk and legs are affected, articles of clothing or detergents are often the agents. And, when the pattern of involvement diffusely involves the entire body, an airborne allergen, pollen or gas, is the likely offender.

Assuming the sensitizer is recognized and subsequent exposure is prevented, the contact dermatitis it caused will gradually clear in ten to twenty days. Continuing exposure, however, will result in chronic dermatitis with dark thickened skin in varying degrees of irritation.

Can contact dermatitis be prevented?
It is not always possible to prevent contact dermatitis, because no one knows exactly what plants, chemical, cosmetics, or household products will cause a reaction. However, once a substance is incriminated, it should never be brought in contact with the skin again. Although some people say they are so allergic to poison ivy that all they have to do is look at a plant and they break out in a rash, this is simply not true. It is the contact that counts and, if the contact is eliminated, the dermatitis will not develop.

Are the weeping sores of contact dermatitis contagious?
No. Not only aren't the sores contagious, they will not even cause an additional reaction on the same person. It is the allergen sensitizer that causes the rash, nothing else. Upon

exposure to the sensitizer, it is possible to increase the areas of sensitization by rubbing or scratching different parts of the body, thus spreading the allergen. However, this can only occur when the allergen is present on the body surface. Once it enters the skin, combines with skin protein, and sets up an allergic response, additional spread is impossible unless additional exposure occurs.

How can an allergen sensitizer be eliminated once contact has been made? And how can it be avoided when its identity is known?

If contact with a known allergen occurs, the area of exposure should be washed with soap and water as soon as possible. By removing the sensitizer from the skin, many reactions can be prevented. Further contact can be avoided by discarding all offensive substances and by having all poisonous plants, trees, and shrubs removed from your surroundings. Also, wearing gloves, boots, and other outer clothing and covering the skin with talc during periods of possible exposure will reduce the chances of reactions taking place.

How can an allergen sensitizer be eliminated when its identity is unknown?

This may seem to be a difficult task, but it is entirely feasible. Whenever contact dermatitis develops and the allergen is not known, every possible sensitizer must be avoided. Isolation is the only means to achieve this objective. The sufferer must totally restrict his or her activities by staying in a "clean" environment, such as a bedroom or hospital. He should dress in only those clothes that have been worn successfully in the past, assuming that they have been washed in a previously tolerated detergent. All cosmetics and grooming aids are forbidden. Windows and doors are to be kept closed, and traveling outside the room is, of course, completely taboo. If the dermatitis does not clear when good isolation is maintained, the offensive substance has been overlooked. But, the search is now limited to the small isolated environment, and the allergen will soon become apparent. If the dermatitis does clear, restrictions can be lifted gradually until normal daily activity is resumed or another attack of dermatitis intervenes. However, this time the rash can be attributed to the last day's exposure, and the allergen can be readily pinpointed.

What constitutes proper therapy for allergic dermatitis?

Local treatment constitutes proper therapy for contact allergic dermatitis. During the early stages of illness, cool sodium bicarbonate or aluminum acetate soaks, thirty minutes three times a day, will reduce inflammation. Large blisters can be sterilely punctured with a needle, and the thin deflated skin should be allowed to remain intact over the naked blister base. (As mentioned previously, the blister fluid is neither infectious nor contagious.) Soothing lotions can be applied as needed to lessen itch and diminish irritation.

For severe reactions, bed rest is advised.

What are the most effective ingredients in OTC lotions and creams?

There are four chief ingredients in contact dermatitis medications.

Antihistamines: The antihistamines found in OTC products include diphenhydramine, methapyrilene, and pyrilamine. Each of these drugs counteracts the effects of histamine on blood vessels and also helps to reduce the itching that is attributed to histamine release. Although these drugs are usually tolerated well, they may occasionally cause allergic reactions themselves.

Antiseptics: Antiseptics are intended to restrict the bacteria population at the site of their application and thus reduce the possibility of developing an infection. Present in OTC products for contact dermatitis are such antiseptics as alcohol, phenol, hydrogen peroxide, benzalkonium chloride, and benzethonium chloride. Although each of these substances is effective in limiting bacterial growth, their action is very short lived. In addition, they provide no relief of allergic symptoms like swelling, burning, or itching.

Astringents: These substances cause contraction of swollen tissue, limit bleeding, and reduce inflammation. When used on contact-dermatitis rash, they will slow oozing and relieve irritation. Aluminum acetate, zinc oxide, tannic acid, calamine, and zirconium oxide are found in various OTC products.

Local anesthetics: Benzocaine, dibucaine, tetracaine, cyclomethycaine, diperodon, and pramoxine are individually present in the contact-dermatitis lotions, creams and sprays. They all deaden nerve endings, so the itchy discomfort of allergic sores will not be felt. Unfortunately, for them to be effective they must be present in greater concentrations than are found in the OTC products. Also, they may cause moderate to severe allergic reactions in susceptible people.

RECOMMENDED TREATMENT
A product that contains an antihistamine and an astringent is best suited for the relief of symptoms of contact dermatitis. It should be used in combination with cool water soaks and may be applied at night for comfort while sleeping.

COMMENTS AND CAUTIONS
Remember that before any lotion or cream is applied to the sores, a thorough washing with soap and water is absolutely essential to remove any allergen present on the skin. You should do this immediately after contacting a potential allergen or as soon as you detect the developing dermatitis. Then you can apply the OTC medication of your choice to achieve relief from itching, burning, or other physical discomfort. If the condition does not clear in three weeks, or if it becomes worse, see your doctor.

POISON IVY AND POISON OAK REMEDIES
Boldface: Recommended

Anti-Itch, lotion	benzocaine
	dibucaine
	tetracaine

Blueboro Bath | aluminum sulfate
calcium acetate
boric acid
blue #1

Caladryl, spray | diphenhydramine hydrochloride 1%
calamine
camphor 0.1%
isopropyl alcohol 10%

Caladryl, lotion | diphenhydramine hydrochloride 1%
calamine
camphor 0.1%
alcohol 2%

Caladryl, cream | diphenhydramine hydrochloride 1%
camphor 0.1%
calamine

Calamatum,
ointment, lotion,
spray | benzocaine 3%
calamine
zinc oxide
camphor
phenol

CZO, lotion | calamine 1.95 g/30 ml
zinc oxide 0.95 g/30 ml
glycerin

Dalicote, lotion | diperodon hydrochloride 0.25%
pyrilamine maleate
zinc oxide
camphor
dimethyl polysiloxane
silicone

Dermapax, lotion | pyrilamine maleate 0.22%
methapyrilene hydrochloride 0.22%
chlorpheniramine maleate 0.06%
chlorobutanol 1%
benzyl alcohol 1%
isopropyl alcohol 40%

Didelamine, gel | tripelennamine hydrochloride
methapyrilene hydrochloride
menthol
benzalkonium chloride

Domeboro, bath   aluminum sulfate
calcium acetate

Dome-Paste   zinc oxide gelatin
calamine

Dri Toxen, cream   methapyrilene hydrochloride 1%
zinc oxide 10%
menthol 0.5%
phenol 1%
zinc sulfate 0.5%
greaseless base

Hista-A-Balm,
medicated lotion   diperodon hydrochloride 0.25%
phenyltoloxamine dihydrogen citrate
   0.75%
camphor
menthol
benzalkonium chloride 0.1%

Hista-Calma, lotion   phenyltoloxamine dihydrogen citrate 1%
benzocaine 1%
calamine

Ivarest, cream,
lotion   pyrilamine maleate 1.5%
benzocaine 1%
calamine 10%
camphor 0.3%
menthol 0.7%
zirconium oxide 4%

Ivy Dry, cream   benzocaine
tannic acid 8%
camphor
menthol
methylparaben
propylparaben
isopropyl alcohol

Lanacane, cream   benzocaine
resorcinol

Neoxyn, solution   hydrogen peroxide 2.85%
benzethonium chloride 0.26%
acetic acid 1.15%
propylparaben 0.02%
acetanilide 0.0169%

Nupercainal, cream	dibucaine 0.5% acetone sodium bisulfite 0.37%
Nupercainal, ointment	dibucaine 1% acetone sodium bisulfite 0.5%
Nupercainal, spray	dibucaine 0.25% alcohol 46%
Obtundia Calamine, cream	calamine zinc oxide cresol-camphor complex
Peterson's, ointment	zinc oxide 6.60% tannic acid 2.20% camphor 3.88% phenol 2.50% beeswax 4% lavender oil petrolatum
Poison Ivy Cream	pyrilamine maleate benzocaine 2.5% povidone zirconium oxide 4%
Poison Ivy Spray	benzocaine 0.5% calamine 2% zinc oxide 1% camphor menthol isopropyl alcohol 0.44%
Pontocaine, cream	tetracaine hydrochloride 1%
Pontocaine, ointment	tetracaine base 0.5% menthol 0.5%
Pyribenzamine Cream	tripelennamine 2% water base
Pyribenzamine Ointment	tripelennamine 2% petrolatum
Resinol, lotion	calamine resorcimol zinc oxide

Rhuli, cream	benzocaine 1% camphor 0.3% menthol 0.7% zirconium oxide 1% isopropyl alcohol 8.8%
Rhuligel, gel	camphor 0.3% menthol 0.3% benzyl alcohol 2% alcohol 31%
Rhulihist, lotion	tripelennamine 1% benzocaine 1% calamine 3% camphor 0.1% menthol 0.1% zirconium oxide 1% methylparaben 0.08% propylparaben 0.02%
Rhuli, spray	benzocaine 0.98% calamine 0.98% zirconium oxide 1% camphor 0.098% menthol 0.009% isopropyl alcohol 0.5%
Soyaloid, bath	soy protein polyvinyl pyrrolidone
Surfadil, cream	methapyrilene hydrochloride 2% cyclomethycaine 0.5%
Surfadil, lotion	methapyrilene hydrochloride 2% cyclomethycaine 0.5% titanium dioxide 5%
Topic, gel	camphor menthol benzyl alcohol 9% isopropyl alcohol 30%
Tronothane Hydrochloride, cream, jelly	pramoxine hydrochloride water base

Tyrohist, cream   pyrilamine maleate
                         benzocaine
                         neocalamine
                         camphor
                         menthol
                         benzalkonium chloride

Ziradryl, lotion   diphenhydramine hydrochloride 2%
                         zinc oxide 2%
                         camphor 0.1%
                         alcohol 2%

Zotox, spray   benzocaine
                         calamine
                         zinc oxide
                         camphor
                         menthol
                         isopropyl alcohol

11. Cuts, Scrapes, and Scratches

What are the dangers of cuts, scrapes, and scratches?
The primary danger of a large cut or wound is the immediate blood loss. This is especially true when larger blood vessels are injured along with the skin and underlying tissues. Consequently, prompt first aid and rapid medical assistance are an absolute requirement in such cases.

Otherwise, for lesser cuts, scrapes, and scratches, where bleeding is slight and easily controlled, infection becomes the primary danger that must be prevented.

When do infections occur?
Whereas most of the bacteria found on the body surface are harmless and never cause infection, other bacteria will produce illness if given the chance. The occasion rises when a cut or bruise develops on the skin and the body's first line of defense is broken. During this period, aggressive bacteria will immediately contaminate the wound and utilize the blood and damaged tissues for food. They can reproduce rapidly and grow into large numbers, thus producing infection. Other factors that influence the development of infection include the specific type and number of bacteria present, the degree of injury, personal susceptibility, and general health.

Are bacteria present only during periods of infection?
No. Bacteria constantly live on the skin of humans and all other animals. They usually reside, reproduce, and grow within hair shafts, around the nose and mouth, in the ears, and any place else on the body that provides a suitable habitat. Some bacteria spend their entire lives on the skin.

Others just use the human body as a vehicle to carry them from one place to another. Most of the bacteria that reside on the skin are perfectly harmless and at times even prove beneficial. Only a small number actually cause human infections.

What are the common superficial infections?

There are several common bacterial infections of the skin.

Cellulitis: Cellulitis is a superficial cellular infection that is caused by strep and staph bacteria. Characterized by soft, swollen sores that become red, warm, and tender, this common ailment usually does not drain, nor does it crust or open. It remains boggy and either expands concentrically or spreads via lymph channels that can be seen as small red lines extending from the sore. The sores may arise anywhere on the body.

Furuncles and *carbuncles:* A furuncle, or boil, is a small abscess that forms at the base of a hair follicle where it also involves, and possibly destroys, the adjacent sweat and sebaceous glands. It usually appears as a tender, firm, red bump that may or may not come to a head and then drain. When several furuncles join under the skin, the larger resultant sores are called carbuncles. These may also "point" and drain pus and blood. Staph bacteria are usually the cause of furuncles and carbuncles.

Folliculitis: Similar to furuncles, but much more superficial and insignificant, folliculitis is an inflammation and infection of hair follicles. Unlike furuncles, no involvement of sweat or sebaceous glands occurs. Rather, very small, painless pustules develop where a hair shaft extends from the skin surface. Itching may be the most annoying symptom.

If this condition persists, freshly formed pimples may be associated with older ruptured sores that are small, red, and encrusted. Again, staph is usually the offending bacteria in cases of folliculitis.

Impetigo: Impetigo is the most superficial of all the bacterial skin infections. It is caused by staph and strep bacteria and usually begins very quickly as a small reddish yellow blister that itches but rarely causes pain. Ultimately, the blister will pop, and a loose, scaly, red brown crust will form over the open, red sores, that are usually round and can measure up to an inch in diameter. These sores may occasionally touch.

Ecthyma: Ecthyma is a deeper form of impetigo caused by the same two bacteria. It occurs most frequently on the legs and begins as a large pustule that ruptures, leaving a pus-covered base with a ragged red margin. Eventually, the entire sore will encrust but, if the crusts are removed, the ulcerated base will be noted to contain and produce more pus.

Paronychia: This infection of the fingernail generally begins as a small break or tear in the cuticle and goes on to produce swelling, redness, pus, and pain along the side of the nail. Ultimately, if the infection is left untreated, the nail growth will be affected, and deformed fingernails will result.

Intertrigo: When infection develops in skin folds, especially in the summer, as a result of perspiration, irritation, and chafing, intertrigo is probably present. Obese people are primarily affected because fatty skin tends to fold easily and provides the warmth and moisture that is conducive to the staph and strep growth that causes this ailment. The affected skin is red, itchy, and slightly tender. With continued irritation, the skin may actually peel off leaving open, inflamed patches that burn and ooze.

External ear infections: external ear infections result when irritations in the external ear canal become invaded with disease-causing bacteria. If only peeling, flaking, redness, and pain are present, infection is unlikely, but when pus is noted a true infection exists.

Minor cuts, abrasions, and burns: Whenever the skin is injured, the possibility of superficial infection markedly increases. The causative bacteria will most likely be those already present on the skin at the time of the injury, but infection can occur later if the appropriate germs are introduced. The most common infectious agents of cuts and abrasions are staph and strep bacteria.

How are the different superficial infections treated?
Depending on the nature and extent of infection, treatment
will vary. Here are some suggestions:

Cellulitis: Rest, local heat applied through warm wet
compresses, and antibiotics are recommended. If topical antibiotics in the form of creams, lotions, or ointments prove
ineffective, prescription drugs taken by mouth are indicated,
and a doctor must be consulted.

Furuncles and carbuncles: By applying warm, wet heat to
furuncles and carbuncles, these deeper abscesses may come
to a head and drain spontaneously. Sometimes they will
simply go away on their own. Larger abscesses frequently
require surgical drainage that is most properly conducted by
a physician.

Since furuncles and carbuncles are relatively deep, local
antibiotics have little effect because they cannot penetrate
the deeper skin tissues. However, when drainage occurs,
topical antibiotics can be used around the sores to prevent
contamination and infection of adjacent skin and hair follicles.

Folliculitis: This condition is best treated by frequent
washings with soapy water and maintenance of good skin
hygiene. Pustules may be gently opened, then washed thoroughly. Antibiotic creams and lotions may be used.

Impetigo: These skin lesions should be washed frequently
with soap and water or a mild hydrogen peroxide solution, so
all loose scales are removed. Then, a topical antibiotic
should be applied to any and all sores, infected or not.
Extensive cases, especially in children, require prescription
antibiotics and professional medical care. Isolation of the
infected individual is also very important because impetigo is
a highly contagious disease.

Ecthyma: Ecthyma should be treated like impetigo.

Paronychia: Successful self-treatment of paronychia can
be achieved if conscientious therapy is quickly initiated and
followed to completion. At the first signs of infection, swelling, tenderness, and redness along the side of the nail, soaking the affected finger in hot saltwater for twenty minutes at

least three times a day will provide soothing relief of pain and limitation of infection. Then, a topical antibiotic should be gently applied to the affected area, and a loose bandage can be used as a dressing. Therapy should continue until evidence of infection is gone. If infection does persist, see a doctor.

Intertrigo: Initial chafing without ulceration may simply be treated with talcum powder, and every attempt must be made to keep the skin folds apart and well aerated. If open sores develop, a topical antibiotic cream or lotion should be applied after the area is well cleansed with a mild soapy solution. Gauze pads, not cotton, can be placed between the folds as dressings that will allow airing and prevent the continued abrasive effect of skin rubbing against skin.

External ear infections: See Treatment, Chapter 18, "Earaches," (pages 208-09).

Minor cuts, abrasions, and burns: Immediately following a cut, scrape, or burn, the injured skin should be washed thoroughly with soapy water in an attempt to eliminate any bacteria that might be present in or around the injured tissue. Topical antibiotics can be used on cuts and scrapes, but they are not necessary. Tincture of iodine, alcohol, merthiolate, or other likely antiseptics and a bandage will ordinarily suffice. Burns with blisters or open, oozing patches should receive topical antibiotic treatment and a light gauze protective covering. For additional information about burns, refer to Chapter 6, "Burns" (pages 46-50).

What antiseptics are available without a prescription? Just about every antiseptic can be bought without a prescription. The more common forms include alcohol; iodine compounds and solutions; oxidizing agents, like hydrogen peroxide; and metal compounds, such as silver nitrate and phenyl mercury. In 1974, the Federal Drug Administration recognized the following antiseptics as safe and effective: benzalkonium chloride, benzethonium chloride, hexylresorcinol, methylbenzethonium chloride, and tincture of iodine. These can be found in a variety of OTC products.

What antibiotics are available without a prescription?
Bacitracin, gramicidin, neomycin, tetracycline, and polymyxin B are all available without a prescription and come in
creams, lotions, and ointments intended for topical use.
Generally, they are equally effective against a wide variety
of bacteria and frequently are marketed as combination
products.

The rationale behind combination products resides in the
fact that some bacteria are resistant to some antibiotics and
by blending two or more antibiotics in one medication,
effectiveness is more or less guaranteed.

RECOMMENDED TREATMENT
I see no great advantage of one antiseptic over another.
The least expensive product should work as well as the
most expensive product.

Although I usually do not favor combination products,
I advocate the use of topical combination antibiotics,
especially those containing bacitracin, neomycin, and
polymyxin B. These products are well established and
proven effective.

COMMENTS AND CAUTIONS
If any of the superficial infections becomes extensive,
spreads rapidly, or begins to penetrate deeper tissue, self-
treatment is not advisable. A doctor should be consulted.

Cuts that bleed extensively, pump blood, injure nerves,
or puncture deeply into the hands or feet must also be
treated by a doctor.

Sutures are usually required if the edges of a laceration
cannot be brought together or if damaged tissue extends
up out of the wound. Deep puncture wounds should always be examined by a physician, regardless of location. A
tetanus shot might be needed.

ANTIBIOTIC CREAMS AND OINTMENTS
Boldface: Recommended

Achromycin,
ointment

tetracycline hydrochloride 3%

Aureomycin,
ointment

chlortetracycline 3%

Baciguent, ointment

bacitracin 500 units/1 g

Baximin, ointment

polymyxin B sulfate 5000 units/1 g
bacitracin 400 units/1 g
neomycin sulfate 5 mg/1 g

**Bacimycin,
ointment**

bacitracin zinc 500 units
neomycin sulfate 3.5 mg

Myciguent, cream,
ointment

neomycin sulfate 5 mg/1 g

**Mycitracin,
ointment**

polymyxin B sulfate 5000 units/1 g
bacitracin 500 units/1 g
neomycin sulfate 5 mg/1 g

**Neo-Polycin,
ointment**

polymyxin B sulfate 5000 units/1 g
bacitracin zinc 400 units/1 g
neomycin sulfate 3.5 mg

**Neosporin,
ointment**

polymyxin B sulfate 5000 units/1 g
bacitracin zinc 400 units/1 g
neomycin sulfate 5 mg/1 g
petrolatum

Polycin, ointment

polymyxin B sulfate 8000 units/1 g
bacitracin zinc 400 units/1 g

Polysporin, ointment

polymyxin B sulfate 10000 units/1 g
bacitracin zinc 500 units/1 g
petrolatum

Spectrocin, ointment

neomycin 2.5 mg/1 g
gramicidin 0.25 mg/1 g

Terramycin,
ointment with
polymyxin B sulfate

oxytetracycline hydrochloride 30 mg/1 g
polymyxin B sulfate 10000 units/1 g

**Triple Antibiotic
ointment**

polymyxin B sulfate 5000 units/1 g
bacitracin 400 units/1 g
neomycin sulfate 5 mg/1 g

12. Dandruff

Is dandruff an abnormal condition?
No, not really. Dandruff simply refers to flaking of the scalp,
which is actually a part of normal skin function. As old skin
cells are replaced by new cells, they are shed from the body
surface. This process occurs continuously all over the body
and is completely natural. But because the scalp is covered
with hair, flakes of old cells cannot leave the skin surface
freely. Instead, they become trapped among the hair shafts,
where they can be seen as small white scales. Although the
condition is perfectly normal, it is occasionally unsightly,
especially for those people who have rapidly growing skin.

Why doesn't dandruff occur in children?
Dandruff does occur in children, but it is very uncommon
before the age of five. Between ten and twenty years of age,
it is more frequently noted, affecting approximately 50 percent of the males and females in that age group. After age
twenty, the condition becomes less common and by age
thirty, only about 40 percent of men and women have
noticeable dandruff. Because of the age distribution, it is felt
that secondary sex hormones play a role in accelerated skin
shedding and excessive flaking of the scalp.

**Is dandruff the only scalp condition that results in
noticeable flaking and scaling?**
No, psoriasis and seborrhea are two other common scalp
conditions that result in unsightly flaking and scaling.

**How can you tell the difference between dandruff and
these other two conditions?**
Dandruff is a simple uncomplicated problem. It is associated
with small white scalp flakes. But seborrhea and psoriasis

have other more serious components. Both of these conditions give rise to larger, coarser flakes along with redness and irritation of the scalp. Furthermore, they not only occur on the scalp, they may also be found on other parts of the body, namely the face, elbows, knees, chest, back, and pubis. By comparison, simple dandruff should only occur on the scalp.

Can dandruff be controlled?

Dandruff can be controlled by using OTC products that are available for this problem. These products contain a wide variety of ingredients that work in different ways but have a similar overall effect: less noticeable scalp flaking. The ingredients for OTC dandruff medications fall into three major groupings.

Resorcinal, salicylic acid, sulfur: By reducing the size of danduff scales and facilitating their removal from the scalp, resorcinol, salicylic acid, and sulfur help make dandruff less noticeable. Each of these agents exerts a disruptive effect on keratin, a major protein found in surface skin cells, and, as a result of this action, the cells are loosened from the scalp, then broken down into smaller, less noticeable fragments. Unfortunately, since hair is also composed of keratin, it may be affected too, becoming dull, brittle, and lifeless. When using these antidandruff agents, care must be taken to avoid contact with the eyes, nose, or mouth because of possible irritation.

Selenium, zinc: Both selenium and zinc decrease the growth rate of skin cells. Because the cells grow slower, they slough slower, and dandruff flaking becomes proportionally reduced. The effectiveness of these elements in controlling dandruff appears to be about the same when they are used in equal concentrations. When applied to already irritated skin or scalp, a slight burning sensation may result.

Coal tar, pine tar, juniper tar: The medicinal tars that are used to treat a number of skin conditions are derived from organic materials such as coal and wood. Associated compounds include anthracene, naphthalene, phenanthrene, phenol, o-cresol, o-xylene, carbazole, toluene, and quinoline. Although these products have undesirable colors and odors, they work well in fragmenting dandruff scales and are used in chronic, difficult dandruff cases. On the negative side, they have been known to cause photosensitivity reactions (sun-related dermatitis) and, because they delay cell growth, they also retard wound healing.

RECOMMENDED TREATMENT
Ordinary dandruff really needs no medical treatment. Simple daily shampooing will remove unsightly flakes. If, however, shampooing is inadequate for you, I suggest a dandruff product that contains zinc or selenium. Since these medications have proven effectiveness and few toxic consequences, they can be used daily and should provide acceptable results. Coal tar products should be reserved for problem dandruff that fails to respond to lesser treatment. They can also be used intermintently in conjunction with a zinc or selenium shampoo, especially when the scalp becomes unruly.

COMMENTS AND CAUTIONS
Like so many other medications, dandruff products can become less effective the longer they are used. Our bodies become refractory to the medically active ingredients. If you notice that your scalp becomes insensitive to the dandruff product you use, switch products and ingredients for a short time, following the recommendations of this chapter. Also, be sure to allow the shampoo time to work on your scalp. Before washing the rest of your body, apply the dandruff product, rub it into your scalp and allow it to penetrate. Rinse off the shampoo at the end of your bath or shower. In this way the product will be more effective.

DANDRUFF OR SEBORRHEA MEDICATIONS
Boldface: Recommended

Anti-Dandruff	Zinc pyrithione 0.1%
Brylcreem, shampoo	mineral oil
	propylene glycol
	paraffin wax
	water

Breck One, cream, zinc pyrithione 1.0%
lotion, shampoo surface active cleansers 15.6%

Dalex, shampoo zinc pyrithione 1.0%
surface active cleansers

Dandricide, rinse isopropyl alcohol
benzalkonium chloride
lauryl isoquinolinium bromide
polysorbate 80
sorbitol

Dandricide, shampoo triethanolamine
lauryl sulfate
propylene glycol
sodium undecylenic monoethanolamido-
  sulfosuccinate
laneth-10 acetate
linoleamide diethanolamine
hydrolyzed animal protein
imidazolidinylurea
methyparaben
propylparaben

Danex, shampoo zinc pyrithione 1.0%
sodium methylcocoyl taurate
magnesium aluminum silicate
sodium cocoyl isethionate
citric acid
fragrance

Diasporal, cream salicylic acid 2%
sulfur 3%
isopropyl alcohol 95%

Flex, antidandruff zinc pyrithione
shampoo

Fomac, cream salicylic acid 2%
cleanser sulfur 2%
detergents

Head & Shoulders, zinc pyrithione 2%
cream shampoo detergent

Head & Shoulders,   zinc pyrithione 2%
lotion shampoo   lauryl sulfate
                           cocamide
                           ethanolamine
                           triethanolamine
                           magnesium aluminum silicate
                           hydroxypropyl methylcellulose

Ionil, shampoo   salicylic acid 2%
                           polyoxyethylene ethers
                           benzalkonium chloride 0.2%
                           alcohol 12%

Klaron, lotion   salicylic acid 2%
                           sulfur 5%
                           alcohol 13.1%

Long Aid Sulphur,   salicylic acid 0.89%
ointment   sulfur 0.89%

Metasep   parachlorometaxylenol 2%
                           isopropyl alcohol 6%

Meted, shampoo   salicylic acid 2%
                           sulfur 3%
                           detergents

Meted 2, shampoo   salicylic acid 1%
                           sulfur 2.3%
                           detergents

Monique Dandruff   benzalkonium chloride
Control, shampoo,   alkylisoquinolinium bromide
rinse

Neomark, lotion   salicylic acid 1.6%
                           resorcinol monoacetate 1%
                           coal tar solution 2%
                           betanapthol 1%
                           castor oil
                           isopropyl alcohol 68%

Neutrogena Solid   fatty acids
Soap, shampoo   glycerin
                           olive oil
                           hydrolyzed protein
                           surface active cleansers

Ogilvie, shampoo

disodium monounderylenamide
   sulfosuccinate

pHisoDan, shampoo

salicylic acid 0.5%
sulfur 5%
entsufon sodium
lanolin
cholesterols
petrolatum

Resorcitate, lotion

salicylic acid 1.5%
resorcinol monoacetate 1.5%
alcohol 66%

Resorcitate With
Oil, lotion

salicylic acid 1.5%
resorcinol monoacetate 1.5%
castor oil 1.5%
alcohol 81%

Rezamid, tinted
shampoo

resorcinol 2%
sulfur 2%
chloroxylenol 0.5%
alcohol 28.5%
cleanser

Rezamid, tinted
lotion

resorcinol 2%
sulfur 5%
chloroxylenol 0.5%
alcohol 28.5%

Rinse Away, liquid,
gel

benzalkonium chloride 0.12%
lauryl isoquinolinium bromide 0.12%

Scadan, scalp lotion

cetyltrimethylammonium bromide 1%
stearyl dimethyl benzyl ammonium
   chloride 0.1%
aqueous vehicle

Sebaquin, shampoo

diiodohydroxyquin 3%

Sebaveen, shampoo

salicylic acid 2%
sulfur 2%
oatmeal 5%
emollients 4%

Sebb, shampoo

triethanol amine
disodium mono-oleamide sulfosuccinate

Sebisol, shampoo	salicylic acid 2% clorophene 0.1% betanaphthol 1% surface active cleansers aliphatic alcoholamide
Sebucare, shampoo	salicylic acid 2% laureth-4 SD alcohol 40 butyl ether dehydroabietyl alcohol
Sebulex, shampoo	salicylic acid 2% sulfur 2% surface active cleansers wetting agent
Selsun Blue, shampoo	selenium sulfide 1% surface active cleansers
Soltex, shampoo	clorophene 0.1% alkyl-aryl surface active cleansers aliphatic alcoholamide
Suave, dandruff control shampoo	sulfur
Sul-Blue, shampoo	selenium sulfide 1%
Sulfur-8, hair and scalp conditioner, ointment	sulfur 2% menthol 1% triclosan 0.1%
Sulfur-8, shampoo	triclosan 0.2%
Tegrin, medicated shampoo	coal tar allantoin
Thylox PDC, shampoo	zinc sulfide salicylanilide
Vanseb, shampoo	salicylic acid 1% sulfur 2% proteins surface active cleansers
Zincon, shampoo	zinc pyrithione 1% surface active cleansers

13. Diaper Rash and Prickly Heat

What is diaper rash?

Diaper rash is a common inflammation of the skin, a form of dermatitis that occurs beneath the diapers of newborn infants, predominantly between the ages of four months and two years.

Why does it occur?

Some of the reasons for diaper rash are quite obvious. The most important causative factor is the ammonia that is released from the infant's urine in the presence of certain bacteria. As the urine and ammonia are rubbed into the skin by soiled diapers, the rash develops.

The bacteria themselves also contribute to the problem because they not only create more ammonia in the urine, they produce infection as well. Their numbers will increase following a bowel movement if the diapers are not changed and the stool is allowed to remain in contact with the skin for a prolonged period of time. Acid stools that are passed by infants on high-protein formulas will also irritate or burn the skin if extended contact is overlooked. Furthermore, the rubber and plastic pants that are worn over the diapers hold in moisture and promote heat, two factors that favor bacterial growth.

Other causes exist, too. For instance, if a harsh detergent is used to wash the diapers and the diapers are not rinsed properly, residual detergent chemicals will irritate the skin. High room temperatures will promote the diaper dermatitis, too.

What does diaper rash look like?
In mild or early cases, the only sign of irritation will be a slight redness that begins where the skin and diapers have maximum contact. As the condition worsens, tiny blisters may form and subsequently develop into small erosions or large ulcers if the problem is not corrected. Due to the presence of many bacteria, infections at the sites of irritation and ulceration are common and frequently give rise to a foul odor and pus.

What is the expected course of diaper dermatitis?
Although the ailment is generally confined to the pubis, genitals, and buttocks, extension to the abdomen, thighs, and calves is sometimes seen in extreme cases where parental neglect or inexperience delays necessary treatment. When this happens, the general health of the infant is in jeopardy. Generally, however, with proper therapy the condition will clear in a few weeks, but occasionally a particularly persistent rash will last for months, even when parental care is meritorious.

How should the problem be treated?
Since the causes of diaper rash are well established, treatment is fairly straightforward. Diapers must be changed frequently. Adequate bathing of the child is essential. Rubber or plastic pants should be avoided (disposables are ideal). And the nursery room should be kept cool and dry.

When cloth diapers are used, laundering techniques become especially important. Laundry services provide an excellent means of obtaining clean, sterile, cloth diapers that have a low potential to produce diaper rash. If washing is done at home, a quick rinsing by hand to remove stool and urine should precede soaking in an antiseptic solution. Then, the diapers should be machine washed thoroughly with an extended rinse cycle, if possible, and dried completely in a dryer at a maximum heat setting or outside in bright sunlight.

Any existing rashes or sores on the infant require immediate attention. These areas should be kept clean and dry in an attempt to prevent secondary infection. An antibacterial cream or lotion should be gently rubbed into each sore, thereby eliminating harmful bacteria. Once the initial dermatitis is cleared, the use of protective powders and creams will generally reduce the possibility of future irritation.

What is prickly heat?

Prickly heat is another form of dermatitis that commonly affects infants. The small, red, pimple-like sores that characterize this ailment most often arise on the face and neck and in the body folds.

Why does this condition develop?

Prickly heat occurs when sweat gland ducts, that normally carry perspiration to the surface of the body, become obstructed. As the sweat accumulates within the blocked duct, pressure rises until the gland or duct ruptures and the salty perspiration leaks out, causing irritation, inflammation, and swelling of the surrounding tissues.

What factors bring on this ailment?

Anything that increases the body temperature and induces perspiration can bring on prickly heat. Consequently, the problem is worse during the hot, humid days of summer, during periods of illness and fever, or when overdressing the infant results in physical discomfort and sweating.

Can prickly heat be prevented?

For the most part, prickly heat can be prevented by keeping the child cool and comfortable. During the summer, the infant should be dressed lightly and allowed to go naked whenever possible. Air conditioning is usually helpful in that it promotes a cool, dry environment that tends to prevent sweating. When baby is hot and irritated, cool water baths will reduce body heat and provide relief. For added protection, an appropriate cream or lotion may be applied to sensitive susceptible areas.

What medications provide adequate protection against diaper rash and prickly heat?
There are quite a few. Here are the ones that are most widely used.

Boric acid: Boric acid has both antibacterial and antifungal qualities, which make it appropriate for controlling bacterial growth on the skin of newborns. However, toxicity to this acid is now well known in the medical profession, and its use is not recommended.

Benzethonium chloride, benzalkonium chloride: These agents safely and effectively keep bacterial counts low for short periods of time. They provide no protection against skin irritation, however, and must be used in combination with other ingredients to prevent the dermatitis of diaper rash and prickly heat.

Fish liver oil, mineral oil: Fish liver oil and mineral oil provide a thin oily covering for the skin and help to prevent the chafing that initiates the diaper dermatitis and prickly heat. They are both safe for infant use.

Lanolin: Lanolin provides protection similar to that of fish liver oil and mineral oil, but occasionally it produces sensitivity reactions.

Petrolatum: By creating a thick physical barrier between skin and diaper, petrolatum reduces friction and alleviates the abrasion that leads to both forms of infantile dermatitis.

Talc: Talc is another safe and effective protection that can be used to prevent diaper rash and prickly heat. It prevents irritation and chafing and also absorbs offensive moisture as well. Care must be taken, however, to prevent the infant from breathing in the powdered talc products.

Vitamins A and D: The effectiveness of vitamins A and D in preventing infant skin irritation resides in the oils, creams, or lotions that are used to carry these agents. Their individual worth has not been sufficiently documented.

Zinc oxide: Last but not least on the list of diaper rash and prickly heat aids is zinc oxide. This compound has been used for years with excellent results and virtually no ill effects. Not only does it create a physical barrier between skin and diaper, it also has a mild antibacterial action and reduces inflammatory swelling. It is probably the most effective agent that can be used for these minor infant skin problems.

RECOMMENDED TREATMENT
Since the Federal Drug Administration is preparing to restrict the use of boric acid in babies' skin aids, I would advise staying away from this agent even though it is found in several products. On a positive note, I highly recommend zinc oxide, alone or in combination with talc, fish liver oil, mineral oil, or petrolatum,

COMMENTS AND CAUTIONS
Diaper rash and prickly heat, although common everyday infant ailments, may lead to serious skin infections. Consequently, they should be prevented, especially since prevention is an easy task. If for some reason the condition gets out of hand and you notice enlarging sores with pus, bring the child to a doctor. Oral antibiotics may be necessary to clear the infection.

DIAPER RASH AND PRICKLY HEAT MEDICATIONS
Boldface: Recommended

A and D, ointment	fish liver oil petrolatum-lanolin base
Ammens Medicated Powder	zinc oxide 0.10% talc 45.06% starch 41% boric acid 4.55% 8-hydroxyquinoline 0.1% 8-hydroxyquinoline sulfate 0.05% aromatic oils 0.14%
Ammorid Dermatologic Ointment	zinc oxide benzethonium chloride lanolin

Ammorid Diaper Rinse, powder	methylbenzethonium chloride edetate disodium
Aveeno Bar, cleanser	oatmeal 50% soap-free sudsing agent lanolin
Aveeno Colloidal Oatmeal, powder	oatmeal derivatives
Aveeno Oilated, liquid	oatmeal 43% lanolin petrolatum
Bab-Eze Diaper Rash Cream	zinc oxide cod liver oil aluminum acetate balsam of Peru ciperodon hydrochloride 0.25% starch
Baby Magic, lotion	benzalkonium chloride lanolin refined sterols
Baby Magic, oil	mineral oil lanolin
Baby Magic, powder	methylbenzethonium chloride
Baby Ointment	zinc oxide benzoin boric acid aluminum hydroxide balsam tolu phenol lanolin petrolatum
Balmex Baby Powder	zinc oxide talc starch balsam of Peru calcium carbonate

Balmex Medicated Lotion	allantoin balsam of Peru silicone lanolin
Balmex Ointment	zinc oxide vitamins A and D balsam of Peru bismuth subnitrate silicone
B-Balm Baby Ointment	zinc oxide 10% benzoin tincture 0.155 ml/30 g phenol 65 mg/30 g methyl salicylate 20 mg/30 g
Borofax, ointment	boric acid 5% lanolin
Caldesene, medicated ointment	zinc oxide talc cod liver oil lanolin petrolatum
Caldesene, medicated powder	talc calcium undecylenate 10%
Codanol A&D, ointment	vitamin A 1500 units/g vitamin D 200 units/g petrolatum lanolin
Comfortine, ointment	zinc oxide 2% boric acid 2% lanolin vitamins A and D
Comfortine, ointment	zinc oxide vitamins A and D lanolin
Covicone Cream	silicone nitrocellulose castor oil greaseless cream base

Cruex, powder, aerosol powder	talc calcium undecylenate 10%
Dalicreme, cream	diperodon hydrochloride 0.25% methylbenzethonium chloride 0.1% vitamins A and D scented greaseless base
Dalisept, ointment	diperodon hydrochloride 1% methylbenzethonium chloride 0.1% vitamin A 750 units/1 g vitamin D 75 units/1 g hexachlorophene 1% lanolin petrolatum
Desitin, baby powder	talc benzethonium chloride
Desitin, ointment	zinc oxide talc cod liver oil petrolatum lanolin
Diapakare, baby powder	corn starch benzethonium chloride sodium bicarbonate
Diaparene, baby powder	methylbenzethonium chloride 1:1800 corn starch magnesium carbonate
Diaparene, ointment	methylbenzethonium chloride 1:1000 petrolatum glycerin
Diaparene Peri-Anal Creme	cod liver oil methylbenzethonium chloride 1:1000 water repellent base
Diaprex, ointment	zinc oxide zinc stearate boric acid balsam of Peru water resistant base

Johnson & Johnson Medicated Powder	zinc oxide talc menthol fragrance
Johnson's Baby Cream	mineral oil paraffin lanolin beeswax ceresin
Johnson's Baby Powder	talc
Lanolar, lotion	purified lanolin
Mediconet, cloth wipe	benzalkonium chloride 0.02% hamamelis water 50% glycerin 10% ethoxylated lanolin 0.5% methylparaben 0.15% perfume
Methakote Pediatric Cream	talc benzethonium chloride protein hydrohysate
Mexsana Medicated Powder	zinc oxide camphor corn starch triclosan kaolin
Morunguent, ointment	cod liver oil concentrate lanolin petrolatum
Oilatum Soap, cleanser	vegetable oil 7.5%
Panthoderm, cream	dexpanthenol 2% water miscible base
Rexall Baby Powder	talc fragrance

Silicote, cream	dimethicone 30% titanium dioxide 1%
Silicote, ointment	dimethicone 33.3%
Silon, spray	silicone zinc oxide lanolin alcohol cetyl alcohol dextran paraffins
Spectro-Jel, gel	cetylpyridinium chloride 0.1% glycol-polysiloxane 1% isopropyl alcohol 15% methylcellulose 1.5%
Taloin, ointment	zinc oxide calamine methylbenzethonium chloride eucalyptol silicone base
Vaseline Pure Petroleum Jelly	petrolatum 100%
ZBT Baby Powder	talc 95.158% magnesium stearate 1.9% mineral oil 2%
Zincofax, cream	zinc oxide 15% lanolin petrolatum

14. Diarrhea

What is diarrhea?
Diarrhea is the excessive passage of loose, watery, unformed stools or bowel movements that are too frequent and too soft.

What constitutes too frequent or too soft?
Generally, each person has some degree of regularity. One person may have three bowel movements each day while another person may have only one every three days, but each is normal. When a person who has three bowel movements each day begins to have five or six and the stool is loose and watery, diarrhea is likely. Similarly, if the person who experiences only one bowel movement every three days starts to have one or two unformed stools each day, the change is consistent with diarrhea.

What are the causes of diarrhea?
The list of possible causes of diarrhea is very extensive and requires a slight knowledge of the different parts and functions of the intestinal tract for understanding. Let us quickly review some selected intestinal organs and discuss the function of each.

Esophagus: The esophagus is a muscular tube that connects the throat with the stomach. Food is pushed through the esophagus by rhythmic contractions of the esophageal muscles.

Stomach: The stomach is a muscular pouch which is located at the end of the esophagus. Its main functions are as follows:

(1)   The release of acid, pepsin, and other digestive juices.
(2)   The mixing of food with the digestive juices of the stomach by muscular contractions and pulsations.
(3)   The absorption of water, sugar, and other substances.
(4)   The moving of partially digested food into the intestines.

Duodenum: The duodenum is the first part of the small intestine. It, too, is a muscular tube which, at one end, is attached to the stomach and, at the other end, joins the jejunum—the second part of the small intestine. The primary functions of the duodenum are as follows:
(1)   Additional mixing of food and digestive juices.
(2)   Absorption of digested food stuffs and water.
(3)   Passage of food along the intestinal tract.

Pancreas: The pancreas is a gland which makes enzymes. These pancreatic enzymes are specific digestive juices needed to break fats, proteins, and carbohydrates into small units that can be absorbed from the intestines. Flowing through a small tube, these enzymes empty into the duodenum where they are mixed with the food already present there.

Gallbladder: Bile, which is manufactured in the liver, is stored and released from the gallbladder. It, too, flows into the duodenum through a small tube leading from the gallbladder and aids in fat digestion.

Jejunum: The jejunum comprises the second part of the small intestine and, like the duodenum that precedes it and the ileum that follows it, is a hollow muscular tube. The jejunum performs the following functions:
(1)   Secretion of additional digestive juices.
(2)   Continued mixing of food with these juices.
(3)   Absorption of digested material and water
(4)   Passage of food into the ileum.

Ileum: The third and final portion of the small intestine, the ileum, has the same functions as the jejunum, only it leads into the large intestine. In all, from the beginning of the duodeum to the end of the ileum, about eighteen feet of small intestine mix, move, digest, and absorb food.

Large intestine: The large intestine is divided into several portions (cecum, ascending colon, transverse colon, descending colon, and sigmoid colon), but each has similar functions. Generally, they include the following:

(1) Secretion of mucus to aid in the passage of waste material into the rectum.
(2) Continued digestion of small fragments of food by millions of bacteria that normally populate the large intestine
(3) Absorption of water and other substances making for more solid intestinal waste.
(4) Passage of the waste materials of digestion on to the rectum.

Rectum: The rectum is a sac where intestinal waste collects until it is eliminated from the body with a bowel movement. Since the rectum is also a muscular tube, it can contract in waves and push feces (waste products of digestion) out of the body.

What causes diarrhea?
Generally, diarrhea results when excessive fluids enter the intestine or when the absorption of the fluid normally present in the intestines is inadequate. Both of these conditions result in rapid movement of food through the bowel and frequent watery bowel movements.

What are the specific causes of this rapid movement?
There are seven major causes of diarrhea.

Irritation: Irritation of the gastrointestinal tract can result in diarrhea by stimulating the muscles that are found within the walls of the intestines. Once stimulated, these muscles contract and propel food rapidly, through the gut. Because of this rapid transit, food and water are not properly digested or absorbed and quickly pass out of the body as loose, poorly formed stools.

Food poisoning, which is due to toxic substances and bacteria present in spoiled or unpreserved foods, is a very common cause of intestinal irritation and diarrhea. Bacteria themselves, along with parasites, frequently cause diarrhea when they are ingested by drinking impure water or by placing contaminated objects in the mouth. Viruses will frequently cause loose watery stools, especially in children, as part of a complex of symptoms common to what doctors call viral gastroenteritis, or intestinal flu.

Drugs, such as some laxatives, will also produce diarrhea through direct irritation of the intestinal walls. Antibiotics which alter the beneficial bacteria that normally live within the intestines can cause diarrhea. Other drugs, such as medications for high blood pressure, sometimes act on the nerves which are responsible for the regular contractions and pulsations of the intestines and thus produce diarrhea by altering those contractions.

Emotional factors: Frequent causes of diarrhea are emotional stress and anxiety. These factors can lead to a condition known as spastic colon, a minor but widespread problem accounting for as much as 50 percent of all intestinal disorders. Along with gas, cramps, and occasional constipation, diarrhea is a frequent feature of spastic colon and results from spastic irregular contractions of the large bowel.

Inflammatory disease: There are several serious inflammatory diseases that cause a rather persistent diarrhea. The most common include ulcerative colitis, an inflammation of the large bowel which can be very debilitating and often requires hospitalization, and regional enteritis, a disease of the third portion of the small intestine, the ileum, which also produces severe diarrhea and other serious intestinal symptoms.

Malabsorption: Some people fail to adequtely absorb fats, carbohydrates, proteins, water, vitamins, and minerals from the intestines. Instead, these important nutrients pass rapidly through the bowel and comprise a diarrhea that is common to the malabsorption disorders. Because general malnutrition results from these diseases, many different symptoms, in addition to diarrhea, result. Bleeding problems, muscular pains and cramps, scaly skin, and bone irregularities are just a few of the other more serious complications.

Allergy: Sensitivity to foods and drugs may produce an allergic reaction in the bowel that occasionally leads to diarrhea.

Hormones: There are eight different endocrine glands, small organs that make hormones. Three of these, the adrenal glands, the thyroid gland and the parathyroid glands, can cause diarrhea when they malfunction. The diarrhea is insignificant, however, when compared to the other extreme effects that result from these hormone disorders.

Surgery: Frequently following stomach or intestinal surgery, diarrhea occurs because of rapid bowel emptying and incomplete digestion.

What can be done for diarrhea?

Initially, an attempt should be made to find the cause. For example, if medication is provoking the diarrhea (oral antibiotics, laxatives, or high blood pressure pills), the offensive drug should be discontinued or changed, if possible. Hopefully, this change will correct the problem. If stress or anxiety is the cause of the diarrhea, a change in life-style might prove helpful in restoring regular bowel habits and improving health in general.

For rapid symptomatic relief of sudden diarrhea, numerous over-the-counter antidiarrheal products are available. These agents should be used only when the diarrhea is infrequent and uncomplicated by other more serious physical symptoms. Although OTC products should sufficiently control mild to moderate diarrhea, severe cases are best treated by a physician.

What medications are available without a prescription?

Medications for diarrhea fall into four major groupings.

Absorbent compounds: These products work by absorbing toxins, excessive water, and bacteria from the intestines, thereby reducing bowel irritation and promoting slower and more natural bowel movements. Unfortunately, they also absorb vitamins, nutrients, certain drugs, and other substances that the body either needs or can use.

Generally considered safe, with few frequent adverse reactions, except for possible constipation, these agents are found in many OTC products and can be used by just about anyone. Ingredients include aluminum hydroxide, atta-pulgite, bismuth, charcoal, kaolin, magnesium trisilicate, pectin, and polycarbophil. Bismuth subnitrate products should be avoided, especially in infants, because of possible ill effects on blood pressure and red blood cells.

Anticholinergic drugs: By a direct action on the nerves that regulate intestinal contractions and movements, anti-cholinergic drugs will limit diarrhea by slowing down intesti-nal motion and bowel movements. However, because of the potential hazards of these drugs, their concentration in anti-diarrhea products is limited by law and probably ineffective.

Atropine sulfate, hyoscine hydrobromide, and hyoscy-amine sulfate are the anticholinergic drugs found in over-the-counter antidiarrhea products. These drugs should not be used by children under six years of age or by people with glaucoma.

Lactobacillus: Lactobacilli are bacteria which are nor-mally found within the intestinal tract. Their use as anti-diarrheal agents is intended to control diarrhea produced by antibiotics that disturb the normal bacterial count in the intestines. Taken in pill form or acidophilus milk, the lac-tobacilli will repopulate the bowel and control diarrhea.

Opiates: These are narcotic drugs which have a recognized effect in the control of diarrhea and, when used as directed, they safely and adequately reduce intestinal contractions and bowel movements. Since they are poorly absorbed from the intestinal tract, they do not have noted general effects on the body, and the possibility of addiction is insignificant. The opiates found in OTC antidiarrheal products, opium and paregoric, are available in some states while other states restrict their sale.

RECOMMENDED TREATMENT
For mild cases of diarrhea, I believe a mixture of kaolin and pectin should sufficiently control the problem. OTC products containing opium or paregoric, along with kaolin and pectin, are more effective and can be used for moder-ate cases if state law permits sales.

COMMENTS AND CAUTIONS

Diarrhea is a frequent disorder that everyone experiences at one time or another and, for the most part, it is an annoyance rather than a disability. However, diarrhea can be a signal of serious intestinal disturbances. Therefore, it is not recommended that antidiarrhea medication be taken for more than two days if the problem persists and, when the diarrhea is associated with additional physical problems, a visit to the doctor is in order. Those problems, occasionally associated with diarrhea, that should arouse concern and a physician's evaluation include nausea, vomiting, bloating, bloody bowel movements, and persistent diarrhea with mucus and streaks of blood.

Because an excessive amount of water is lost from the body with diarrhea, it is important to replace that fluid by drinking clear liquids. Sudden bouts of diarrhea can be combated with the wise selection of an OTC medication and fluid foods taken in small quantities. Solid food can slowly replace fluid meals as bowel movements become less frequent and stools become firmer.

Children, especially the very young, are extremely sensitive to fluid loss. When diarrhea in an infant is present for more than twelve hours, or is complicated by vomiting, call the doctor.

ANTIDIARRHEAL MEDICATIONS
Boldface: Recommended

Amogel, tablet	kaolin 120 mg pectin 15 mg bismuth subgallate 120 mg opium 1.2 mg zinc phenolsulfonate 15 mg
Bacid, tablet	carboxymethylcellulose sodium 100 mg lactobacillus acidophilus

Bisilad, suspension

kaolin 11 g/30 ml
bismuth subgallate 300 mg/30 ml
eucalyptus oil
methyl salicylate
thymol
menthol

Cams, tablet

lactobacillus acidophilus

Corrective Mixture,
liquid

bismuth subsalicylate 480 mg/30 ml
pepsin 240 mg/30 ml
phenyl salicylate 120 mg/30 ml
zinc phenolsulfonate 60 mg/30 ml
alcohol 1.5%

Corrective Mixture
with Paregoric,
liquid

bismuth subsalicylate 480 mg/30 ml
pepsin 240 mg/30 ml
phenyl salicylate 120 mg/30 ml
zinc phenolsulfonate 60 mg/30 ml
paregoric 3.6 ml/30 ml
alcohol 2%

Diabismul,
suspension

kaolin 5 g/30 ml
pectin 160 mg/30 ml
opium 14 mg/30 ml
methylparaben
propylparaben

DIA-quel, liquid

pectin 144 mg/30 ml
paregoric 4.5 ml/5 ml
homatropine methylbromide 0.75 mg/
   30 ml
alcohol 10%

Digestalin, tablet

bismuth subgallate 3.80 mg
activated charcoal 5.30 mg
pepsin 2 mg
berberis 1.20 mg
papain 1.20 mg
pancreation 0.40 mg
hydrastis 0.08 mg
animal diastate 0.06 mg

Donnagel,
suspension

kaolin 6 g/30 ml
pectin 143 mg/30 ml
sodium benzoate 60 mg/30 ml
hyoscyamine sulfate 0.1037 mg/30 ml
atropine sulfate 0.0194 mg/30 ml
hyoscine hydrobromide 0.0065 mg/30 ml
alcohol 3.8%

Donnagel-PG,
suspension

kaolin 6 g/30 ml
pectin 143 mg/30 ml
powdered opium 24 mg/30 ml
sodium benzoate 60 mg/30 ml
hyoscyamine sulfate 0.1037 mg/30 ml
atropine sulfate 0.0194 mg/30 ml
hyoscine hydrobromide 0.0065 mg/30 ml
alcohol 5%

Infantol Pink, liquid

pectin 223.62 mg/30 ml
bismuth subsalicylate 394.68 mg/30 ml
opium camphorated fluid 0.0468 ml/30 ml
calcium carrageeenan 108 mg/30 ml
zinc phenolsulfonate 105.52 mg/30 ml
saccharin sodium 8.22 mg/30 ml
alcohol 0.0408 ml/30 ml
peppermint oil 0.00468 ml/30 ml

Kalpec, liquid

kaolin 3 g/30 ml
pectin 270 mg/30 ml

Kaolin Pectin
Suspension

kaolin 5.83 g/30 ml
pectin 130 mg/30 ml
saccharin
glycerin
carboxymethylcellulose
flavor

Kaomagma,
suspension

kaolin 6 g/30 ml
alumina gel

Kaopectate,
suspension

kaolin 5.8 g/30 ml
pectin 130 mg/30 ml

Kaopectate
Concentrate,
suspension

kaolin 8.75 g/30 ml
pectin 194 mg/30 ml

Lactinex, tablet

lactobacillus acidophilus
lactobacillus bulgaricus

Pabizol with
Paregoric,
suspension

bismuth subsalicylate 517 mg/30 ml
paregoric 3.69 mg/30 ml
aluminum magnesium silicate 265 mg/
    30 ml
phenyl salicylate 97.4 mg/30 ml
zinc phenolsulfonate 51.8 mg/30 ml
alcohol 8%

Parelixir, liquid

pectin 145 mg/30 ml
tincture of opium 0.2 ml/30 ml
alcohol 18%

Parepectolin,
suspension

kaolin 5 g/30 ml
pectin 162 mg/30 ml
paregoric 3.7 ml/30 ml
alcohol 0.69%

Pargel, suspension

kaolin 6 g/30 ml
pectin 130 mg/30 kl

Pektamalt, liquid

kaolin 6.5 g/30 ml
pectin 600 mg/30 ml

Pepto-Bismol,
tablet, suspension

bismuth subsalicylate
calcium carbonate
aminoacetic acid

Polymagma Plain,
suspension

activated attapulgite 3 g/30 ml
pectin 270 mg/30 ml
alumina gel

Quintess, suspension

activated attapulgite 3 g/30 ml
colloidal attapulgite 900 mg/30 ml

15. Drowsiness and Fatigue

How can drowsiness and fatigue be overcome?
Physical conditioning, whereby the energy reserves of the body are brought to a higher level through running, swimming, walking, or other conditioning exercise, provides an excellent means of delaying fatigue. But even the most conditioned athlete will tire eventually. When this happens, or when we run out of energy ourselves, the best way to regain our ability to work effectively is through rest and sleep, since energy compounds are restored during this time.

What are stimulants?
Stimulants are drugs which excite the central nervous system (brain) and improve alertness, prevent drowsiness, and overcome fatigue.

When should stimulants be used?
As a physician, I must discourage the broad use of stimulants but, being a realistic person, I also understand that there are times when people definitely need an energy boost. Truck drivers with demanding schedules occasionally must drive day and night. Students studying for exams, night watchmen, pilots, doctors, and others who must work long hours might also need mental stimulation to help them through their labors. Although it is certainly better to regain alertness and overcome fatigue with a good night's sleep, occasionally it is impossible to do so. In this circumstance stimulants might prove beneficial.

172

What stimulants are available over the counter?
The only stimulant available over the counter is caffeine.

What is the effect of caffeine on the central nervous system?
Caffeine stimulates all parts of the brain: the cortex, where thought, movement, and sensations originate; the cerebellum, which controls coordination; the medulla, an area that regulates the breathing and heart rate; and, finally, the pons and spinal cord, regions of the brain that contain millions of nerve connections.

What are the effects of caffeine on the heart?
Caffeine has been shown to stimulate heart muscle, thereby increasing the heart rate, magnifying the force of each heartbeat, and generally producing a greater blood flow. Large doses of caffeine may sometimes make the heart beat slightly irregularly.

How effective is caffeine as a stimulant?
This is a question that is open to mixed opinions. Some studies have shown that, although people taking caffeine felt more alert and energetic, their performance on simple tests was no better than that of people who had not taken the drug. Other studies, based on automobile driving and the performance of simple mental tasks, proved that caffeine did improve mental activity, especially when the testing sessions were long, tiring, and boring. Therefore, I personally think that caffeine does act as a mild mental stimulant.

Can the effectiveness of caffeine be increased?
Yes, the effectiveness of caffeine can be increased if it is used infrequently. Like so many drugs, with continual use caffeine may eventually become tolerated by the body, and its effectiveness will decrease. It may be that continued use of the drug allows the body to adjust to its presence, thereby reducing its stimulating effect. With infrequent use, the

body doesn't have a chance to adjust, and caffeine can cause a maximum burst of energy.

Is the use of caffeine associated with any side effects?
Yes. Some people complain of headaches, irritability, sleeplessness, nervousness, anxiety, and jitters when they consume large doses of caffeine.

Since coffee contains caffeine and also causes stomach distress, will caffeine produce the same effects?
Probably not. Although coffee has been shown to significantly increase the release of acid in the stomach, caffeine has not. In fact, decaffeinated coffee, which has no caffeine in it, will produce the same acid-releasing effects as regular coffee. Therefore, it is probably the coffee rather than the caffeine that causes gastric distress.

Can caffeine reduce hangovers?
The notion that caffeine will bring quick relief from hangovers is a popular misconception that has no factual substantiation. However, when this drug is given to someone who is intoxicated, it does help to restore alertness by counteracting the depressant effects of alcohol or sedative drugs.

We know that caffeine is found in coffee, but are there other drinks that also contain this drug?
Yes, there are. Tea and cola soft drinks also contain caffeine. While coffee contains approximately 125 milligrams of caffeine per cup, tea contains about 65 and cola about 40. The caffeine in these beverages will also produce mental stimulation and alertness.

RECOMMENDED TREATMENT
If a stimulant must be taken, I recommend one which contains no ingredients other than caffeine. Wise consumers will look for the least expensive product.

COMMENTS AND CAUTIONS

Caffeine is a safe drug, but overdoses do occur when the drug is greatly misused. Problems can virtually be eliminated if the caffeine is used infrequently and in recommended quantities. Furthermore, it must be remembered that there is no substitute for sleep—a vital body need.

Also consider this: There are times when drowsiness and fatigue are not related to overwork and overexertion. Occasionally, mental problems, such as depression and anxiety, or physical disease, including anemia, low blood sugar, and infection, will weaken and tire the body. Sometimes the fatigue results from serious medical problems like leukemia, thyroid disease, and diabetes. And generalized muscular weakness may be caused by disorders in the nervous system or skeletal muscles. Therefore, if your fatigue is long-standing, and unimproved by rest and sleep, consult your doctor.

STIMULANTS
Boldface: Recommended

Amostat, tablet	caffeine 100 mg
Chargers, capsule	caffeine 100 mg dextrose
Caffedrine, capsule	caffeine 250 mg
Double-E Alertness, capsule	caffeine 180 mg thiamine hydrochloride 5 mg
Nodoz, tablet	caffeine 100 mg
Prolamine, capsule	caffeine 140 mg phenylpropanolamine hydrochloride 35 mg

Quick-Pep, tablet	caffeine 150 mg niacin 10 mg thiamine mononitrate 3 mg
Tirend, tablet	caffeine 100 mg
Verb T.D., capsule	caffeine 200 mg
Vivarin, tablet	caffeine 200 mg dextrose 150 mg
Wakoz, tablet	caffeine 200 mg

16. Dry Skin
(Flaking, cracking, stiffness, and roughness)

Everyone suffers from dry skin occasionally. What causes it?

The list of individual factors leading to dry skin is a lengthy one. Included in it are chemical irritants and drying agents, such as cleansers and solvents; environmental factors, like wind, cold, and low humidity; personal qualities, including nutrition, health, age, and hormone function; plus overall skin characteristics, such as skin thickness and durability. Although these individual factors lead to dry skin, the actual cause appears to be the skin's inability to hold a normal amount of water. With excessive water loss come the prominent features of dry skin: flaking, cracking, stiffness, and roughness.

What normally prevents water loss from our bodies and our skin?

Our bodies are composed primarily of water, 60 percent to be precise, and infants have an even higher percentage. This water would quickly evaporate into the atmosphere were it not for the skin that surrounds and protects the body like a giant flexible container. And what holds moisture in the body's natural covering? Well, the skin essentially protects itself. As skin cells move toward the surface of the body, they flatten and become filled with a protein, called keratin, which makes them firm and durable. When they reach the surface, they die but remain intact for several days, providing a physical barrier that protects the underlying living cells. The retention of water is one of the most important protective functions of these keratinized cells.

Other factors also influence the skin's ability to hold water. The oils that are manufactured by the tiny sebaceous glands, found throughout the skin, provide a film that helps to retain water. Also, a substance, called the natual moisturizing factor, has been recently identified and apparently acts as a chemical sponge that holds fluid within the skin. The natural moisturizing factor may, in fact, be the most important water retainer of all.

What is the composition of the natural moisturizing factor?
Chemical analysis of the natural moisturizing factor has revealed several of its constituents, but complete identification is currently unavailable. To date, urea, sugar, small protein fractions, and numerous other components have been isolated. Apparently, these substances work collectively to maintain the hydration of the keratin layer of the skin and also bind water themselves, thus promoting fluid retention in at least two ways.

What are the features of dry skin?
Dry skin can affect any part of the body but is usually most pronounced on the hands and forearms, feet and lower legs, face and neck—areas of maximum exposure. The skin is generally dry, slightly flaky and often develops crisscross lines that slowly become conspicious over a prolonged period of time. At first, the condition may come and go with the seasons, improving in the summer and relapsing in the winter. However, in time, the symptoms become permanent, and the small flaky patches may grow into larger, more irritated lesions. Itching may occur, but usually it is not severe.

How should dry skin be treated?
The first step in treating dry skin should include a search for any causative factors enhancing the conditions, such as detergents, irritating clothes, chemical solvents, and so forth. Further contact with these agents must be avoided. Room humidification may prove very helpful, especially in the winter when heated homes become exceedingly dry and skin ailments are particularly troublesome. As a rule, fre-

quent bathing only aggravates dry-skin conditions, so they should be restricted as much as possible. When they are necessary, the use of a bath oil will counteract the drying effects of soaps and shampoos. After bathing, a dry-skin lotion should be generally applied to the body with particular emphasis on problem areas.

What are the ingredients in dry-skin lotions, creams, and baths?
Ingredients for these medications fall into six main categories.

Allantoin: Allantoin is found in several dry skin products. It has a softening effect on keratin, the protein that is so abundant in the surface cells of the skin. It also allows water to be replenished in the keratin layer.

Glycerin: Glycerin is a substance that attracts water and, for this reason, is used as a skin moisturizer. However, for it to be effective it must be absorbed into the skin, and this usually doesn't happen. Instead, glycerin will remain on the body surface where it will actually draw additional moisture from already dry skin. Consequently, its use as a moisturizer is questionable.

Oil: In an attempt to duplicate the natural moisture-retaining qualities of oily sebaceous secretions, animal, vegetable, and mineral oils are included in a variety of dry-skin products. When applied to the skin, they form a slick barrier at the surface and help to seal in moisture. Mineral oil is probably the most effective.

Petrolatum: Petrolatum is another physical agent that forms a sealing water barrier on the surface of the skin. It is more effective than any oil and even surpasses silicone in its moisturizing qualities. Unfortunately, petrolatum is messy. Since it is not absorbed, it always leaves the skin feeling greasy and slick; furthermore, it will often stain clothing.

Urea: Urea, like allantoin, softens keratin and allows water to reenter the skin. It has been used successfully to treat dry-skin problems for years and imparts more pliability than allantoin. Since it is one of the components of the natural moisturizing factor, its beneficial qualities become immediately apparent.

Vitamins: Vitamins, A, D, and E are all essential dietary factors required for normal healthy skin and body function, but play no major role in the treatment of dry skin when simply applied to the skin's surface. Although they are found in several skin lotions and creams, their only effect is a mild occlusive action that is better performed by other agents, such as petrolatum or mineral oil.

RECOMMENDED TREATMENT
Any product that contains urea in combination with petrolatum or mineral oil is, in my opinion, the most suited for dry-skin conditions. The presence of glycerin in low concentration can be overlooked. Since vitamins only add to the expense of a dry-skin preparation without providing significant benefits, I see no indications for their use.

COMMENTS AND CAUTIONS
The dry-skin creams and lotions produce few, if any, side effects. Just about the only possibility is an allergic reaction to one of the ingredients (lanolin is incriminated most frequently). If you use a dry-skin lotion, and irritation develops or a rash appears, discontinue usage and switch to another product.

DRY-SKIN MEDICATIONS
Boldface: Recommended

Albolene, cream	mineral oil
	petrolatum
	paraffin
	ceresin
	carotene
Alpha Keri, bath oil	mineral oil
	lanolin oil
	peg-4-dilaurate
	benzophenone-3
	fragrance
	green #6

Aquacare, cream, lotion	urea 2% glycerin oleth-3 phosphate petrolatum triethanolamine synthetic spermaceti carbomer 934P mineral oil lanolin alcohol cetyl stearyl glycol lanolin oil benzyl alcohol perfume
Aquacare/HP, cream, lotion	urea 10% glycerin oleth-3 phosphate cetyl stearyl glycol petrolatum triethanolamine synthetic spermaceti carbomer 934P mineral oil lanolin alcohol lanolin oil benzyl alcohol perfume
Carmol, cream	urea 20% nonlipid base
Carmol Ten, cream	urea 10% nonlipid base
Clocream Ointment	vitamin A vitamin B cream base
Corn Huskers Lotion	glycerin 6.7% alcohol sodium alginate galactomannan

Dermassage, lotion

mineral oil
tea stearate
propylene glycol
stearic acid
diammonium phosphate
methyl paraben
lanolin
triclosan
urea
propylparaben

Domol Bath and
Shower Oil

di-isopropyl sebacate
isopropyl myristate
mineral oil

Domol, lotion

refined mineral oil
purcelline oil, synthetic

Emulave, soap

glycerin
vegetable oils
dewaxed lanolin
colloidal oatmeal

Esoterica, lotion

propylene glycol
dicaprylate
tea stearate
mineral oil
isocetyl stearate
glyceryl stearate
cetyl esters wax
animal protein
dimethicone
tea carbomer 941
methylparaben
propylparaben
quaternium-15

Jergens Direct Aid,
lotion

allantoin
water
sorbitol
stearic acid
coceth-6
glyceryl dilaurate
glyceryl stearate
lard glyceride
stearamide
hydrogenated vegetable oil

isopropyl palmitate
polyethylene glycol 100 stearate
dimethicone
petrolatum
sodium carbomer 941
fragrance
methylparaben
quaternium-15
propylparaben
simethicone

Jergens for Extra
Dry Skin, lotion

allantoin
glycerin
water
coceth-6
glyceryl dilaurate
lard glyceride
mineral oil
isopropyl palmitate
stearic acid
dimethicone
methylparaben
sodium carbomber 941
fragrance
propylparaben
quaternium-15
simethicone

Jergens Hand Cream

allantoin
glycerin
water
stearic acid
alcohol
potassium stearate
propylene glycol dipelargonate
fragrance
lanolin oil
tetrasodium dicarboxyethylstearyl
    sulfosuccinate
potassium carbomber 934
methylparaben
polysorbate 81
simethicone
salicylic acid
cellulose gum
propylparaben

Jeri-Bath, oil	dewaxed lanolin mineral oil emulsifier
Jeri-Lotion	dewaxed lanolin mineral oil emulsifier
Keri Cream	water mineral oil talc sorbitol ceresin lanolin alcohol magnesium stearate glyceryl oleate isopropyl myristate methylparaben propylparaben fragrance bromonitropropandiol
Keri Lotion	mineral oil lanolin oil propylene glycol glyceryl stearate peg-40-stearate peg-4-dilaurate laureth-4 methylparaben propylparaben fragrance carbomer 934 triethanolamine dioctyl sodium sulfosuccinate
Lacticare Lotion	lactic acid 5.0% sodium PCA 2.5% mineral oil isopropyl palmitate coceth-6 sodium hydroxide glyceryl stearate myristyl lactate cetyl alcohol carbomer 940

imidazolidinyl urea
dehydroacetic acid

Lubriderm, cream

glycerin
lanolin derivatives
cetyl alcohol
petrolatum

Lubriderm, lotion

lanolin derivatives
mineral oil
sorbitol
cetyl alcohol
triethanolamine
petrolatum
stearic acid
methylparaben
butylparaben
propylparaben

Milk Plus 6, lotion

propylene glycol
isopropyl myristate
dicaprylate/dicaprate
lanolin
alcohol
tea stearate
almond oil
glyceryl stearate
polysorbate 20
cetcareth-5
dry milk
wheat germ oil
sesame oil
safflower oil
avocado oil
castor oil
spermaceti
dimethicone
tea carbomer

Neutrogena, body oil

isopropyl myristate
sesame oil

Neutrogena, dry-
skin soap

triethanolamine
stearic acid
tallow
glycerin

	coconut oil
	water
	castor oil
	sodium hydroxide
	oleic acid
	laneth-10 acetate
	purcelline oil
	cocamide DEA
	BHT
	o-tolyl biguanide
Neutrogena, hand cream	glycerin
	fatty alcohol sulfate
	stearic acid
	glycinello
Nivea, cream	glycerin 3%
	water
	mineral oil
	waxes
	isopropyl myristate
	fatty alcohol
	lanolin oil
	glycerin monostearate
	wool wax alcohol
	aluminum stearate
	magnesium stearate
	magnesium sulfate
	fragrance
	formaldehyde
Nutraderm, lotion, cream	mineral oil
	aliphatic alcohols
	balanced emulsifiers
Nutraplus, lotion, cream	urea 10%
	glyceryl stearate
	acetylated lanolin
	alcohol
	isopropyl palmitate
Mutraspa, liquid	dewaxed lanolin
	mineral oil
	soapless surfactant
Oil of Olay, lotion	mineral oil
	potassium stearate

sodium stearate
cholesterol
cetyl palmitate
butyl paraben
sodium carbomer 934
potassium carbomer 934
propylparaben
methylparaben
sodium laurate
potassium laurate
castor oil
sodium myristate
potassium myristate
myristal alcohol
sodium palmitate
potassium palmitate
stearyl alcohol

Oilatum, soap   polyunsaturated vegetable oil

Pacquin, lotion,   glycerin
cream   stearic acid
                         potassium stearate
                         sodium stearate
                         myristal lactate
                         cetyl alcohol
                         spermaceti
                         stearamide DEA
                         di-isopropyl sebacate
                         methylparaben
                         propylparaben

Pond's, cold cream   mineral oil
                         isopropyl palmitate
                         sorbitan oleate
                         glycerin
                         lanolin
                         ceresin
                         triethanolamine

Rain Tree, lotion   mineral oil
                         propylene glycol
                         glyceryl stearate
                         stearic acid
                         lanolin oil
                         propyl paraben

	oat flour
	methylparaben
	triethanolamine
Rose Milk, lotion	cetyl alcohol
	glyceryl stearate
	mineral oil
	glycerin
	stearic acid
	sorbitan lanolate
	trietanolamine
	dimethicone
	methylparaben
	propylparaben
Saratoga Ointment	zinc oxide
	boric acid
	eucalyptol
	servum preparatum
	white petrolatum
Sardo, bath oil	mineral oil
	isopropyl myristate
	isopropyl palmitate
Sardoettes, towelettes	mineral oil
	isopropyl myristate
	isopropyl palmitate
Sayman Salve, ointment	propylene glycol
	petrolatum
	zinc oxide
	camphor
	lanolin
Shepard's, lotion	sesame oil
Siliderm, lotion	glycerin
	silicone
	nonsensitizing lanolin
	purified water
	perfume
	sorbic acid
Skin Quencher, lotion	petroleum
	glyceryl stearate
	stearic acid

phenol dimethicone
di-isopropyl adipate
glycereth-26
triethanolamine/laneth 16
choleth-24
carbomer 940
imidazolidimyl urea
methylparaben
propylparaben

Sofenol, lotion

glycerin
peanut oil
lanolin
cetyl alcohol
stearyl alcohol
water
perfume
triethanolamine stearate
sorbic acid

Tega E, cream

vitamin E
cream base

Thilene 4-M, lotion

allantoin 0.25%
cleansers
wetting agents
emulsifiers
dispersants

Tridenol, liquid

olive oil
vegetable oils
surfactant

Triple Lanolin
Lotion

mineral oil
stearic acid
lanolin
sorbitol
ethoxydiglycol
triethanolamine
cetyl alcohol
palmitate
methylparaben
propylparaben

Vaseline Intensive
Care, lotion

glycerin
glyceryl stearate
stearic acid

mineral oil
cetyl alcohol
laureth-23
tri-isopropanolamine
lanolin
isopropyl palmitate
methylparaben
propylene glycol
carbomer-934
propylparaben
simethicone

Wibi, lotion

emulsifying wax
polyglycols
alcohol
menthol
glycerol

Woodbury for Extra
Dry Skin, lotion

allantoin
glycerin
water
alcohol
mineral oil
triethanolamine stearate
stearyl alcohol
lanolin
hydrogenated vegetable oil
cetyl alcohol
sodium carbomer 941
methylparaben
polyparaben
fragrance

17. Dyspepsia
(Indigestion, acid stomach and heartburn)

What are the underlying causes of indigestion, acid stomach and heartburn?
Generally, indigestion, acid stomach and heartburn result from excessive acid in the stomach. The specific causes are listed herein.

Dietary causes: Spicy or poorly cooked foods; eating too much, too little, or too quickly; excessive use of coffee, tea, alcoholic beverages, or tobacco; or stomach-irritating drugs.

Mental causes: Possibly fatigue, anxiety, nervousness, fear, and overwork.

Physical causes: Gastritis, esophagitis, ulcers, and cancer are also associated with the symptoms of gastric distress.

What can be done for indigestion?
First, the underlying cause should be determined and eliminated if possible. This may be quite simple. For example, if heartburn develops every time you drink coffee, common sense should tell you to remove coffee from your diet. If hasty meals bring on indigestion, eating should be slowed down and more relaxed. These problems may become obvious after a little thought and consideration. Anxiety, nervousness, fear, and overwork may be more difficult to recognize and control.

Usually, antacid therapy will provide quick relief of gastric distress regardless of the cause.

What distinguishes physical causes of indigestion from dietary and mental causes?
Dietary and mental causes for indigestion are not usually associated with actual esophagus or stomach damage, while

physical causes always indicate that injury to these digestive organs has taken place. Dietary and mental factors can, however, lead to actual physical disease and frequently do so.

Do the physical causes for indigestion have distinctive symptoms?
Yes and no. Generally, they share common symptoms, but differences can be noted.

Esophagitis: Recurrent heartburn, or pain in the middle of the chest, is the most common symptom of esophagitis and usually occurs after a large meal. The heartburn becomes worse when lying down or bending over and frequently is pronounced at bedtime because of the horizontal position of the body. Belching acidity may also occur, and, occasionally, excessive pain and difficulty in swallowing are experienced.

Another condition that results in esophagitis is hiatal hernia. In this condition, because the stomach and esophagus are insecurely held in place by the diaphragm, acid reflux irritates the esophagus and produces the common complaints of heartburn and dyspepsia.

Gastritis: The symptoms of gastritis can be vague and variable. A sensation of pressure or fullness in the stomach might be noted, along with a feeling of nausea, which may or may not be associated with belching and vomiting. Dull burning pain and stomach discomfort may occur with meals.

Stomach ulcers: Stomach ulcers are characterized by a gnawing pain, present in the upper left portion of the belly, which comes and goes at irregular intervals. Occasionally, this pain may be slightly relieved by eating or may disappear immediately following a meal, but at other times, eating may actually cause the discomfort. Nausea and vomiting are experienced by people who have stomach ulcers, and decreased appetite along with weight loss may take place.

Duodenal ulcers: Typically, the most pronounced symptom of duodenal ulcers is a sharp, steady, gnawing pain located in the mid-to-upper part of the abdomen. The pain usually subsides following a meal, but it returns one to three hours later. Other symptoms are variable, and include bloating, belching, heartburn, nausea, and vomiting.

When should a person attempt to treat gastric distress?
People who infrequently suffer from heartburn, dyspepsia, or indigestion can safely and effectively treat their discomfort with antacid products. However, when constant antacid medication is needed, a doctor should be consulted in an attempt to uncover any serious physical illness.

What are antacids?
Antacids are medications used to neutralize excess acid present within the stomach.

Isn't acid always present within the stomach?
Yes, it is; in fact, it is needed for adequate digestion and is produced and released by special cells (parietal cells) found within the stomach.

What causes the release of acid secretion in the stomach?
When food enters the stomach, a hormone called gastrin is released by other specialized cells lining the inner stomach wall. This hormone then stimulates the parietal cells to discharge their acid into the stomach so that food may be digested.

Are there other substances that cause acid release?
Actually, there are several substances other than gastrin that promote acid secretion in the stomach. These include partially digested proteins, coffee, the alcohol commonly found in whiskey, wine, and beer, and even cigarette smoke.

Why doesn't the acid digest the stomach itself?
This is an interesting question, and the answer proves how marvelous our bodies truly are. The stomach not only secretes acid, it also produces and secretes pepsin, a substance that digests protein. Since acid and pepsin can eat a hole

right through the middle of a thick steak, one might right-fully wonder why they don't normally eat a hole right through the stomach. Well, to be factual, in abnormal situations (ulcers) they sometimes do, but generally, the stomach is able to protect itself.

Throughout the stomach, there are numerous mucus glands and cells which make both a thin watery mucus and a thick sticky mucus which line the interior of the stomach and prevent the acid and the pepsin from digesting the stomach as well as the food.

Why should anyone take antacids to neutralize stomach acid if it is necessary for digestion?

Occasionally, acid will be released into the stomach at the wrong time, perhaps because of the tension of a business meeting or maybe because of the frustration of a traffic jam. Regardless, that excess acid will cause discomfort. At other times, when stomach, esophageal, or duodenal irritations are already present, the acid will intensify the problem by causing further damage. Under these circumstances, it is advisable to use an antacid to neutralize the excessive, unneeded, and sometimes destructive acid secretions.

What are the ingredients in OTC antacid products?

There are primarily four major ingredients that appear in OTC antacid products.

Sodium bicarbonate: Sodium bicarbonate is a very effective and rapidly acting antacid which has been used for years. Unfortunately, it has major drawbacks.

1. It may reduce the stomach acidity too much.
2. The sodium is absorbed from the stomach and may cause serious problems (hypertension) if used frequently.
3. Rebound acidity may occur; that is, although the acid already present within the stomach is neutralized, sodium bicarbonate may stimulate additional acid secretion.

Generally, this antacid product is not recommended by doctors.

Calcium carbonate: Calcium carbonate is another effective antacid, but it, too, has serious unwanted side effects.

1. When calcium carbonate comes in contact with the hydrochloric acid in the stomach, a compound, calcium chloride, is produced. Calcium chloride is readily absorbed from the stomach and, with continued use, can build up within the body. Excessive body calcium may cause kidney and nervous disorders.

2. Calcium carbonate also causes increased acid secretion in the stomach and constipation.

Aluminum: Aluminum antacid products come in several forms such as aluminum hydroxide, aluminum carbonate, aluminum phosphate, and aluminum aminoacetate. All of these compounds demonstrate effectiveness in treating stomach acidity.

Aluminum products have several good points: they do not excessively reduce acidity and they are not significantly absorbed by the stomach. However, they have minor drawbacks, too: constipation can result with continued use and normal phosphate absorption from the intestines is diminished. (The second problem can be reduced by using aluminum phosphate products which deliver more phosphate to the intestines and counteract the decrease in phosphate absorption.)

Magnesium: Magnesium antacid products are also varied and include magnesium oxide, magnesium hydroxide, and magnesium trisilicate. These products definitely prove worthwhile, but they are often associated with diarrhea. As with any antacid product, magnesium may cause kidney problems and, like the other preparations mentioned above, should be cautiously used by people who already have some form of kidney disease.

What are the different forms of antacids which are available over the counter?
Antacids come in tablets, powders, gums, lozenges, and liquids.

Which form is most effective?

The liquid form is generally considered to be the most effective because the antacid compounds present within the liquid suspensions are ground into very small particles; and the smaller the particle size, the more effective the antacid. In order for tablets to be as effective, they must be crushed thoroughly in the mouth and dissolved slowly. Gels which are dried, then redissolved, tend to lose their effectiveness; and powders, which must be mixed with water before use, can be inconvenient.

Are the unnecessary additives present in OTC medications?

Some, not all, of the OTC antacids contain compounds which have absolutely no ability to neutralize acid and, in my opinion, should not be used. For example, some antacids contain pain killers, sedatives, anesthetics, antispasmodics, and numerous other drugs that can lead to other potential medical problems when used frequently.

Some antacids contain simethicone. What is this?

Simethicone, a compound contained in several antacid products, has no antacid activity per se, but it does aid in reducing gas and will prove helpful if taken specifically for that purpose.

RECOMMENDED TREATMENT

Combinations of magnesium and aluminum compounds are very effective and safe. Since the aluminum products occasionally cause constipation and the magnesium products are associated with diarrhea, a combination which contains both aluminum and magnesium tends to have offsetting qualities. Also, I prefer liquid suspensions over tablets, gels, gums, and powders. In addition, low sodium preparations are desirable.

COMMENTS AND CAUTIONS

Always bear in mind that illnesses requiring antacid therapy may be as simple as indigestion caused by overeating or as serious as cancer. Therefore, it is imperative to use antacid products wisely. If relief of gastric distress does not occur within two weeks following the start of self-medication, or if blood is noted in vomiting or bowel movements, a doctor should be notified.

In addition, antacids may reduce the effectiveness of iron tonics, digoxin, tetracycline, anticholinergic drugs, chlorpromazine, isoniazid, phenobarbital, nitrofurantoin, penicillin, sulfonamides, and salicylates. And, they may increase the potential of quinine, coumadin, morphine, pseudoephedrine, and quinidine. If you are taking any of the above drugs or any other medication, consultation with a physician is advised before antacids are used.

Since many antacids contain a high concentration of sodium, read the labels of these products before buying them. Choose the one with the lowest sodium content, especially if you are on a low sodium diet or have high blood pressure.

ANTACID MEDICATIONS
Boldface: Recommended

Alkalade, tablet   dihydroxyaluminum aminoacetate 200 mg

Alkalade Plus,   aluminum hydroxide 200 mg/5 ml
suspension   magnesium hydroxide 200 mg/5 ml
                                  simethicone 30 mg/5 ml

Alka-2 Chewable   calcium carbonate 500 mg
Antacid, tablet

Alka-Seltzer   sodium bicarbonate 1000 mg
Effervescent Antacid   citric acid 800 mg
                                  potassium bicarbonate 300 mg

Alkets, tablet	magnesium hydroxide 65 mg calcium carbonate 750 mg magnesium carbonate 130 mg
Aludrox, tablet	aluminum hydroxide 233 mg magnesium hydroxide 84 mg
Aludrox, suspension	aluminum hydroxide 307 mg/5 ml magnesium hydroxide 103 mg/5 ml
Alurex, tablet	aluminum hydroxide magnesium hydroxide
Alurex, suspension	aluminum hydroxide magnesium hydroxide
Aluscop, capsule	magnesium hydroxide 180 mg dihydroxyaluminum acetate 325 mg
Aluscop, suspension	aluminum hydroxide 150 mg magnesium hydroxide 150 mg/5 ml dihydroxyaluminum acetate 200 mg/5 ml methylparaben 0.15%
Amitone, tablet	calcium carbonate 350 mg mint flavor
Amphojel, tablet	aluminum hydroxide 300 mg
Amphojel, suspension	aluminum hydroxide 320 mg/5 ml
A.M.T., tablet	aluminum hydroxide 164 mg magnesium trisilicate 250 mg
A.M.T., suspension	aluminum hydroxide 305 mg/5 ml magnesium trisilicate 625 mg/5 ml
Antacid Powder	aluminum hydroxide 15% magnesium trisilicate 31% sodium bicarbonate 25% magnesium carbonate 10%

Anti-Acid No. 1, tablet	calcium carbonate 227.5 mg magnesium carbonate 130 mg bismuth subnitrate 32.5 mg flavor
Banacid, tablet	aluminum hydroxide magnesium hydroxide magnesium trisilicate
Basaljel, suspension	alumiunum hydroxide 400 mg/5 ml
Basaljel, capsule	aluminum hydroxide 500 mg
Basaljel, tablet	aluminum hydroxide 500 mg
Basaljel Extra Strength, suspension	aluminum hydroxide 1.0 g/5 ml
Bell-Ans, tablet	sodium bicarbonate 264 mg or 527 mg wintergreen ginger charcoal
Bisodol, tablet	magnesium hydroxide 180 mg calcium carbonate 195 mg
Bisodol, powder	sodium bicarbonate magnesium carbonate peppermint oil
Camalox, suspension	aluminum hydroxide 225 mg/5 ml magnesium hydroxide 200 mg/5 ml calcium carbonate 250 mg/5 ml
Camalox, tablet	aluminum hydroxide 225 mg magnesium hydroxide 200 mg calcium carbonate 250 mg
Chooz, gum	magnesium trisilicate 268 mg calcium carbonate 360 mg
Citrocarbonate, suspension	sodium bicarbonate 780 mg/3.9 g sodium citrate 182 g/3.9 g
Citrocarbonate, powder	sodium bicarbonate 106 g/5.1 g sodium citrate 1.33 g/5.1 g

Creamalin, tablet aluminum hydroxide 248 mg
magnesium hydroxide 75 mg
flavor

Delcid, suspension aluminum hydroxide 600 mg/5 ml
magnesium hydroxide 665 mg/5 ml

Dialume, tablet aluminum hydroxide 500 mg

Diatrol, tablet calcium carbonate
pectin
sodium bicarbonate

Dicarbosil, tablet calcium carbonate 500 mg
peppermint oil

Di-Gel, tablet aluminum hydroxide 282 mg
magnesium hydroxide 85 mg
simethicone 25 mg

Di-Gel, suspension aluminum hydroxide 282 mg/5 ml
magnesium hydroxide 87 mg/5 ml
simethicone 25 mg/5 ml

Ducon, tablet calcium carbonate

Eno, powder sodium bicarbonate 7.6%
sodium tartrate 65.2%
sodium citrate 27.2%

Equilet calcium carbonate 500 mg

Estomul-M, aluminum hydroxide 918 mg/5 ml
suspension

Estomul-M, tablet aluminum hydroxide 500 mg
magnesium oxide 45 mg
magnesium carbonate

Fizrin, powder sodium bicarbonate 1825 mg/packet
aspirin 325 mg/packet
sodium carbonate 400 mg/packet
citric acid 1448.5 mg/packet

Flacid, tablet aluminum hydroxide
magnesium hydroxide 85 mg
simethicone 25 mg
magnesium carbonate 282 mg

Gaviscon, tablet dried aluminum hydroxide gel 80 mg
magnesium trisilicate 20 mg
sodium bicarbonate 70 mg
alginic acid 200 mg

Gelumina, tablet aluminum hydroxide 250 mg
magnesium trisilicate 500 mg
sorbitol 18.8 mg
lactose
saccharin sodium

Gelusil, suspension aluminum hydroxide 200 mg/5 ml
magnesium trisilicate 200 mg/5 ml
simethicone 25 mg/5 ml

Gelusil, tablet aluminum hydroxide 200 mg
magnesium trisilicate 200 mg
simethicone 25

Gelusil Flavor-Pack, aluminum hydroxide 250 mg/5 ml
suspension magnesium trisilicate 500 mg/5 ml
flavor

Gelusil-Lac, powder aluminum hydroxide 1 g/packet
magnesium trisilicate 2 g/packet
milk solids

Gelusil M, aluminum hydroxide 250 mg/5 ml
suspension magnesium hydroxide 100 mg/5 ml
magnesium trisilicate 500 mg/5 ml
flavor

Gelusil M, tablet aluminum hydroxide 250 mg
magnesium hydroxide 100 mg
magnesium trisilicate 500 mg
mannitol
flavor

Glycate, tablet calcium carbonate 300 mg
glycine 150 mg

Glycogel, tablet

calcium carbonate 325 mg
aluminum hydroxide 175 mg
magnesium carbonate

Gustalac, tablet

calcium carbonate 300 mg
milk powder 200 mg

**Kessadrox,
suspension**

aluminum hydroxide 1.0 g/15 ml
magnesium hydroxide 165 mg/15 ml
peppermint oil
sorbitol

Kolantyl, gel

aluminum hydroxide 150 mg/5 ml
magnesium hydroxide 150 mg/5 ml

Kolantyl, tablet

aluminum hydroxide 300 mg
magnesium oxide 185 mg

Kolantyl, wafer

aluminum hydroxide 185 mg
magnesium hydroxide 170 mg

Krem, tablet

calcium carbonate 400 mg
magnesium carbonate 200 mg
milk powder 500 mg
flavor

**Kudrox,
suspension**

aluminum hydroxide 565 mg/5 ml
magnesium hydroxide 180 mg/5 ml
sorbitol 1 ml/5 ml

Kudrox, tablet

aluminum hydroxide 400 mg
magnesium carbonate

**Liquid Antacid,
suspension**

aluminum hydroxide 1.0 g/15 ml
magnesium hydroxide 165 mg/15 ml
sorbitol
peppermint oil

**Maalox,
suspension**

aluminum hydroxide 225 mg/5 ml
magnesium hydroxide 200 mg/5 ml

Maalox #1, tablet

aluminum hydroxide 200 mg
magnesium hydroxide 200 mg

Maalox #2, tablet

aluminum hydroxide 400 mg
magnesium hydroxide 400 mg

Maalox Plus,
suspension

aluminum hydroxide 225 mg/5 ml
magnesium hydroxide 200 mg/5 ml
simethicone 25 mg/5 ml

Maalox Plus,
tablet

aluminum hydroxide 200 mg
magnesium hydroxide 200 mg
simethicone 25 mg

Magna Gel,
suspension

aluminum hydroxide
magnesium hydroxide
flavor

Magnatril,
suspension

aluminum hydroxide 260 mg/5 ml
magnesium hydroxide 130 mg/5 ml
magnesium trisilicate 260 mg/5 ml

Magnatril, tablet

aluminum hydroxide 260 mg
magnesium hydroxide 130 mg
magnesium trisilicate 454 mg

Magnesia and
Alumina Oral
Suspension

aluminum oxide 72 mg/30 ml
magnesium hydroxide 124 g/30 ml
sorbitol
saccharin
peppermint

Malcogel, suspension

aluminum hydroxide 330 mg/5 ml
magnesium trisilicate 660 mg/5 ml

Marblen, suspension

aluminum hydroxide
magnesium trisilicate
calcium carbonate
magnesium carbonate
flavor

Marblen, tablet

aluminum hydroxide
magnesiun trisilicate
calcium carbonate
magnesium carbonate
flavor

Maxamag,
suspension

aluminum hydroxide
magnesium hydroxide

Mint-O-Mag, liquid	magnesium hydroxide 390 mg/5 ml sodium carboxymethylcellulose sodium citrate saccharin sodium
Mylanta, suspension	aluminum hydroxide 200 mg/5 ml magnesium hydroxide 200 mg/5 ml simethicone 20 mg/5 ml
Mylanta, tablet	aluminum hydroxide 200 mg magnesium hydroxide 200 mg simethicone 20 mg
Mylanta II, suspension	aluminum hydroxide 400 mg/5 ml magnesium hydroxide 400 mg/5 ml simethicone 30 mg/5 ml
Mylanta II, tablet	aluminum hydroxide 400 mg magnesium hydroxide 400 mg simethicone 30 mg
Neosort Plus, tablet	dried aluminum hydroxide gel 300 mg magnesium hydroxide 150 mg
Nephrox Suspension	aluminum hydroxide 320 mg mineral oil 10%
Neutralox, tablet	aluminum hydroxide 300 mg magnesium hydroxide 150 mg
Noralac, tablet	aluminum hydroxide 300 mg magnesium trisilicate 100 mg bismuth aluminate 100 mg alginic acid 50 mg
Nutrajel, suspension	aluminum hydroxide 300 mg/5 ml
Nutramag, suspension	aluminum oxide magnesium hydroxide
Pama, tablet	aluminum hydroxide 270 mg magnesium trisilicate 260 mg
Phillips Milk of Magnesia, suspension	magnesium hydroxide 2.27–2.62 g/30 ml peppermint oil 1.166 mg/30 ml

Phillips Milk of Magnesia, tablet	magnesium hydroxide 300 mg peppermint oil 1.166 mg
Phosphaljel, suspension	aluminum phosphate 233 mg
Ratio, tablet	calcium carbonate 400 mg magnesium carbonate 50 mg
Riopan, suspension	magaldrate 400 mg/5 ml
Riopan, tablet	magaldrate 400 mg
Robalate, tablet	dihydroxyaluminum aminoacetate 500 mg
Rolaids, tablet	dihydroxyaluminum sodium carbonate 334 mg
Salcedrox, tablet	aluminum hydroxide 120 mg sodium salicylate 300 mg calcium ascorbate 60 mg calcium carbonate 60 mg
Silain-Gel, suspension	aluminum hydroxide 282 mg/5 ml magnesium hydroxide 85 mg/5 ml simethicone 25 mg/5 ml
Silain-Gel, tablet	aluminum hydroxide 282 mg magnesium hydroxide 85 mg simethicone 25 mg magnesium carbonate
Soda Mint, tablet	sodium bicarbonate 324 mg peppermint oil
Spastosed, tablet	calcium carbonate 226 mg magnesium carbonate 162 mg
Syntrogel, tablet	aluminum hydroxide 38% magnesium hydroxide 14% magnesium carbonate
Titralac, suspension	calcium carbonate 1 g/5 ml glycine 300 mg/5 ml

Titralac, tablet	calcium carbonate 420 mg glycine 180 mg
Trimagel, tablet	aluminum hydroxide 250 mg magnesium trisilicate 500 mg
Trisogel, suspension	aluminum hydroxide 150 mg/5 ml magnesium trisilicate 583 mg/5 ml
Trisogel, capsule	aluminum hydroxide 100 mg magnesium trisilicate 300 mg
Tums, tablet	calcium carbonate 500 mg peppermint oil
Wingel, suspension	aluminum hydroxide 180 mg/5 ml magnesium hydroxide 160 mg/5 ml
Wingel, tablet	aluminum hydroxide 180 mg magnesium hydroxide 160 mg

18. Earaches

What causes earaches?
Infections are the leading cause of earaches. They may be
bacterial or viral and occur outside the eardrum in the outer
ear or inside the eardrum in the middle and inner ear.
Regardless of where they originate, pain is a common
symptom.

External ear infections can be quickly identified. An irritated area that is red and swollen, the drainage of pus, a foul
odor, or itching are common findings that indicate external
infections.

Internal infections are much more difficult to self-evalu-
ate. These may follow a cold or flu, or they might arise
without any previous illness at all. The pain is usually severe
and unremitting. Children under five are most commonly
affected.

Other symptoms that relate to middle and inner infections
include fever, dizziness, nausea, vomiting, hearing loss, and
occasionally diarrhea.

If the eardrum ruptures, relief from pain will be dramatic
as pus, blood, and debris flow out the ear canal, but hearing
loss may be permanent and the infection may persist.

Are there other causes of earaches besides infections?
Yes, there are. Trauma to the ear will certainly cause pain
and may result in cuts and bruises. Hematomas, which are
sacular collections of blood within or around the outer ear,
may also occur.

Severe trauma may actually produce a fracture in the

boney wall of the ear canal or possibly puncture the eardrum. Both conditions lead to sudden, severe pain.

Foreign articles that are caught in the ear, or even the buildup of wax within the ear canal, will cause discomfort.

Low on the list, but certainly the most serious cause of pain in the ear, are growths and tumors. Although these are rare, they may produce pain, especially in the outer ear, when they exert pressure on the ear canal. Tumors of the inner and middle ear will create hearing loss, dizziness, and trouble with balance, before they generate pain.

Why do some earaches occur on airplanes?
The Eustachian tube is a small channel that leads from the middle ear to the back of the throat. If this tube is blocked, pressure will increase within the middle ear, and as the plane changes altitude, pain will be noted. The same thing happens to scuba divers.

If the Eustachian tube is open, pressure equalization between the middle ear and the surrounding environment will occur by simply swallowing or holding the nose closed and blowing. Unfortunately, some people are born with narrow Eustachian tubes and will always have trouble "clearing the ears." Others may experience this difficulty only when they have a cold or flu.

RECOMMENDED TREATMENT
Mild earaches that occur with colds and flus may be self-medicated with pain relievers, such as aspirin or acetaminophen, and decongestants. Decongestants will also help to prevent ear stuffiness and discomfort while traveling.

External ear infections should be treated with an antibiotic cream or ointment and mild pain relievers.

COMMENTS AND CAUTIONS
Attempting to self-medicate more serious forms of earaches is foolhardy; frequently it results in permanent ear

damage and hearing loss because proper therapy is delayed.

If signs of a middle or inner ear infection are present, see your doctor immediately. This advice also applies to suspected fractures of the boney ear and perforation of the eardrum.

Foreign obstacles lodged in the ear may be gently removed at home, if they are *easily accessible* with a pair of tweezers. Deeply lodged material should be referred to the doctor.

External ear infections that fail to respond to therapy within ten days should be brought to the attention of a physician.

DECONGESTANT MEDICATIONS

For a listing of decongestants, please turn to Chapter 7, "Colds and Flus" (pages 84-98).

ANTIBIOTIC CREAMS AND OINTMENTS

For a listing of these antibiotics, please turn to Chapter 11, "Cuts, Scrapes, and Scratches" (pages 143-44).

MILD PAIN RELIEVERS

For a listing of these pain relievers, please turn to Chapter 1, "Aches and Pains" (pages 6-14).

19. Fever

How does the body maintain a constant temperature?
Within the brain, in a special center called the hypothalamus, there is a group of nerve cells that constantly
monitor body temperature. When the body becomes over-
heated and the blood flowing through the hypothalamus
becomes warmer than 98.6°, special mechanisms are activated to reduce the temperature. Sweating begins, and, as
the perspiration evaporates, the body becomes cooler. In
addition, blood vessels in the skin enlarge many times, and
warmer blood from deep within the body rushes to the body
surface where it loses heat.

If the body is too cold, opposite reactions take place.
Blood vessels in the skin become smaller, forcing blood to
collect within the warmer internal organs. Perspiration
ceases, and shivering, which occurs as rapid short muscular
contractions, generates heat through increased muscular activity. In this way, the body becomes warmer.

**How can fever occur if the body has a special tempera-
ture-control center in the brain?**
The temperature-control center in the brain, the hypothalamus, has a built-in thermostat, which is normally set at
about 98.6°. When the body becomes invaded by bacteria or
other infectious agents, "fever producers" called pyrogens
are released into the blood stream and are carried to all
parts of the body, including the hypothalamus. These pyrogens alter the temperature-control center by readjusting the
thermostat to a higher setting, and the hypothalamus re-

sponds accordingly to maintain the body at an abnormally high temperature, thus producing a fever.

What can happen to the body if a fever gets too high?
Generally, the body is able to cope with a mild temperature elevation of one to five degrees. However, when a fever reaches 105° convulsions occasionally occur, especially in children. Brain damage will result if a fever of 106° is maintained for a prolonged period of time, and death is common when body temperatures reach 110°.

What are some of the more common conditions that produce fever?
Infections, especially colds, are by far the most common causes of fever. Other less common but more serious causes include leukemias, cancers, blood diseases, blood clots, strokes, brain tumors, and rheumatoid diseases, just to name a few. Generally, with more serious illness, a fever is prolonged and may go up and down in conjunction with other disease symptoms.

What are the characteristcs of a fever?
You don't need a thermometer to know you are ill. Elevated body temperature can frequently be recognized by a sensation of increased warmth on the skin. Headaches and backaches, along with muscular and joint aches and pains, occasionally accompany a fever. And chills, which alternate with an uncomfortable feeling of warmth, also indicate that a fever is present. Although you don't need a thermometer to tell you have a fever, you should use one anyway. Thermometers were one of the first mechanical means of determining illness, and they still prove exceptionally useful today.

Are there any nonprescription drugs that reduce fever?
Yes. Aspirin, phenacetin, acetaminophen, and salicylamide are the most effective antifever drugs, and each is available without a prescription.

How do these drugs work to reduce fever?
Their precise mechanism is not known. Some studies indicate that they increase perspiration and body cooling through evaporation. Other studies demonstrate a direct action on the temperature regulating center in the brain. They may also prevent the release of pyrogens (the temperature-elevating proteins that circulate in the blood during times of infection and tissue damage). Regardless of the precise mechanism, they work.

RECOMMENDED TREATMENT
For control of fever, aspirin or acetaminophen are most widely recommended. Therapy must be continuous, with particular emphasis on afternoon and evening doses, because temperatures normally reach their highest levels at these times. For most adults, 600-700 mg of either aspirin or acetaminophen, every three to four hours, should be sufficient. The dosage for children varies according to age and product selection, so manufacturer recommendations should be followed. Fever therapy should also include constant fluid replacement, in both the adult and child, because dehydration usually results from elevated body temperatures.

Whenever fever in a child is associated with breathing difficulty, stiff neck, rash, or lassitude and stupor, consult your doctor immediately. Monitor a baby's temperature frequently.

COMMENTS AND CAUTIONS
Aspirin and acetaminophen are the most effective antifever medications available with or without a prescription. Although both are safe drugs, each is associated with specific side effects and contraindications, which are reviewed in detail in Chapter 1 of this book (pages 5-6).

ANTIFEVER MEDICATIONS

For a listing of these medications, please turn to Mild Pain
Relievers in Chapter 1, "Aches and Pains" (pages 6-14).

20. Fever Blisters and Cold Sores

What are fever blisters and cold sores?
Fever blisters and cold sores are painful eruptions that occur on the lips, chin, and other parts of the body. They are caused by a virus, herpes simplex, that usually remains dormant in small nerve cells until activated by changes in body environment.

What specific changes activate herpes virus?
Fever and the common cold both lead to herpes activation and subsequent "fever blisters" or "cold sores." The precise mechanism for the activation is unknown, but the painful unsightly sores are well recognized. Other factors, such as exposure to sunlight, hormone changes associated with menstruation, emotional episodes, and fatigue or poor health are also related to outbreaks of herpes infection.

Who is affected by herpes simplex virus and the fever blisters and cold sores that the virus produces?
Just about everyone, with the exception of most newborn babies, is affected by herpes virus. Generally, the virus lives within human cells for prolonged periods of time with no apparent effect on the human host. Then, when activated by one of the factors mentioned above, the virus is propelled into a reproductive state, which results in the disruption and destruction of human cells and the development of a viral sore.

Although almost 100 percent of all adults harbor the herpes virus, only about 30 percent will suffer from recurrent fever blisters and cold sores. Evidently, the recurrent sufferer is unable to develop the proper immunity to keep the virus in check and, consequently, faces the dismal future of continued outbreaks.

Why are newborn babies spared?
As the baby develops in the mother's womb, protective antibodies that the mother has made throughout her lifetime pass through the placenta to the fetus. When the infant is born, these maternal antibodies protect it against disease until the child can manufacture antibodies of its own. Between the ages of one and five, 70 to 90 percent of all children become infected by the herpes virus and, at that time, must produce more antibodies to fight the infection and harness the virus. Those children who successfully meet the viral challenge will probably remain symptom-free for the rest of their lives, but those who fail to respond adequately will suffer from recurrent eruptions in the form of fever blisters and cold sores.

What are the manifestations of herpes viral infections?
During the initial stage of a fever blister or cold sore, a tingling sensation, a burning, or an itch will commence. This is followed within two to four days by a group of tiny blisters that contain clear, colorless fluid and develop where the lip and the skin of the face meet. The blisters will go on to burst, and the sore that remains may bleed or simply become crusted. Soon a scab forms, and within three to fourteen days the lesion heals.

What can be done for fever blisters and cold sores?
Several nonprescription products are available for the treatment of fever blisters and cold sores. They include one or more of the following ingredients:

Aminobenzoate: Aminobenzoate, in various forms, is found in some fever-blister products and is intended to block the ultraviolet rays of the sun, which are known to activate herpes virus. The medication is safe and effective.

Allantoin: Allantoin has a softening effect on the skin and is marketed as a skin moisturizer. However, no known effect on herpes virus is reported.

Benzalkonium chloride: An antiseptic which is safe and effective against bacteria, benzalkonium chloride has no substantiated antiviral activity. When used on fever blisters, it might help to prevent secondary bacterial infections, but secondary infections of fever blisters and cold sores is unlikely, even without the use of an antiseptic or antibiotic.

Camphor, menthol, phenol, tannic acid: These agents exert a mild drying effect and produce temporary numbing of the sore. However, no significant effect against herpes virus has been reported, except possibly for phenol which inhibits viral activity when used in higher concentration in laboratory procedures.

Benzocaine and other anesthetics: Local anesthetics, including benzocaine, dull nerve endings and prevent painful sensations. Although they reduce the discomfort of fever blisters and cold sores, they have no antiviral actions.

Pyridoxine: Pyridoxine acts as a coenzyme in the metabolism of amino acids. Its antiviral activity is questionable, but users report relief.

Lactobacillus acidophilus: Lactobacillus acidophilus is a bacteria found in milk and milk products. It has been used to treat various illnesses and is marketed in the form of tablets and powders for relief of fever blisters and cold sores. The mechanism of action is an increase in the enzyme acid phosphatase, that is found in saliva following ingestion of the bacteria. The phosphatase is said to inhibit herpes virus.

RECOMMENDED TREATMENT

Claims for relief from cold sores are poorly documented by manufacturers, and personal accounts vary. Here's what I suggest.

To soften the sore and promote healing, warm water should be gently applied with a clean washcloth or fragment of gauze or cotton. This procedure should be repeated as frequently as possible during the acute, painful stages of the eruption. In addition, the application of a fever blister and cold sore remedy that contains phenol and camphor in a soothing oil or emollient base should then be administered. Lactobacillus acidophilus might also be tried—if it works, great!

Whenever prolonged sun exposure is anticipated, a sunscreen should be applied to the lips. In this way, the fever blister or cold sore might be totally avoided.

COMMENTS AND CAUTIONS

Please keep this in mind. If the eruption on your lip is painless or persists for more than three weeks, it is probably not a fever blister or cold sore. And, if additional lesions develop elsewhere on your body at the same time, you most likely have a more serious problem. In these circumstances, I would urge you to see your doctor.

FEVER BLISTER AND COLD SORE REMEDIES

Boldface: Recommended

Anbusol, liquid

alcohol 70%
benzocaine
phenol
iodine

Blistex, lip ointment

ammonia
camphor
phenol
petrolatum
mineral oil
lanolin
paraffin
sorbitol
alcohol
sesquioleate
soya sterol
peppermint oil

CamphoPhenique, liquid

camphor 10.8%
phenol 4.7%
aromatic oil solution

Chap Stick, stick
ointment

camphor
petrolatum
lipids
amylparadimethylaminobenzoate

Cold Sore Lotion

benzoin Siam
benzoic acid
chlorothymol
camphor
alcohol 90%

Herpecin, stick
cream

sesame oil
paraffin
octyldodecanol
titanium dioxide
white petrolatum
beeswax
pyridoxine hydrochloride
propyl-p-aminobenzoate
spermaceti
amyldimethyl-p-aminobenzoate
allantoin

Lactinex, tablet

lactobacillus acidophilus
lactobacillus bulgaricus

Tanac, liquid, stick

tannic acid
camphor
menthol
allantoin
benzoamylparadimethylaminobenzoate
benzalkonium chloride
emollients

Vaseline Cold Sore
Medication, stick

camphor ice

21. Fungal Infections of the Skin
(Athlete's foot, ringworm, and jock itch)

What is a fungus?
A fungus is a primitive plant that grows without leaves, roots, or stems. Starting from a seed spore, the fungus first sprouts a single microscopic filament that resembles a bamboo shoot. This filament then divides and grows and divides again until a large branching network has formed. Food is derived from the decomposition of other living organisms, and reproduction is generally accomplished through new spore formation and additional seedings.

How are humans involved with these strange plants?
Fungi, like bacteria, cause infection. They grow both in and on human beings and have the ability to utilize human tissues for food. Generally, the diseases they cause are more disquieting than disabling, but occasionally severe internal infections result in death, especially in debilitated people who have other major medical problems.

Because internal fungal infections are uncommon ailments that require extensive medical management, they will not be discussed in this chapter. Instead, a description of the superficial fungal infections will be presented along with methods of therapy.

Where are skin fungi usually found?
Causing diseases with such descriptive names as "athlete's foot," "jock itch," and "ringworm," the skin fungi have lived in very close association with man for eons. They are found everywhere in nature from field and pond to house and garden, but one of their favorite habitats is human skin.

Although infection does not always occur, the fungi will use people as a vehicle to carry them to the ends of the earth or simply to the backyard swimming pool, where they will await a more susceptible subject.

If a fungus is going to produce an infection, how does it begin?

Fungi invade the surface of the body, including hair, nails, and skin. Because their incubation period is brief, only a few days are required for their spores to germinate within hair follicles, along the edge of fingernails and toenails, or in the most superficial layer of the skin, the stratum corneum. A mass of fungal filaments quickly develops at the site of contact and entangles the hair shaft, grows into the nails, or spreads radially in the skin. Within weeks, a rich growth of fungi disrupts and digests the protein, keratin, which is a major constituent of hair, nails, and skin. You literally become the fertilizer of these skin fungi; and the sweat glands, that are so abundantly dispersed throughout your skin, provide the irrigation for the fungal crop.

If some people develop infections and others don't, what factors determine susceptibility?

To be infected, a person must first come in contact with fungal spores or growing fungal organisms. Since the fungi are found everywhere in nature, contact is easily made. However, direct contact with normal healthy skin rarely produces infection; therefore, other factors must come into play. If an individual has poor hygiene, for example, infection is more likely. General health and nutrition play a significant role, too, since unhealthy people suffer from fungal diseases much more readily than healthy people. Finally, environment influences the possibility of contracting infection. Because the heat and moisture common to tropical and subtropical climates are conducive to fungal growth, living in warmer locations increases the chances of infection.

Fungal infections usually occur on specific areas of the body and are named accordingly. What are the various infections?

Fungal infections of the scalp (Tinea capitis): Tinea capitis is the name given to fungal infections of the scalp which are widespread and, at times, attain epidemic proportions. Children are most commonly affected, particularly boys, but infection generally clears without treatment with the advent of puberty. Those infections that do persist into adult life carry with them the common symptoms of scaling, itching, and inflammation of the scalp. Patchy hair loss may also occur.

Serving as a link between infected and uninfected individuals are such common items as barbers' clippers and combs. The slight scalp irritation that these instruments produce is ideal for the implantation of fungal spores and the initiation of infection.

Fungal infections of the body ("ringworm" or Tinea corporis): Ringworm of the skin, not including scalp, beard, hands, feet, or groin, are given the medical name Tinea corporis. While extremely variable in appearance, the manifestations of bodily fungal infections are obvious. Ranging from classic ringworm sores to collections of small, red, fluid-filled blisters or from deep-seated, hard, multiple nodules to soft, boggy, inflamed patches, infected areas reflect different fungal growth patterns and varied human responses.

The classic ringworm lesions typically develop as small doughnutlike sores that expand concentrically on the skin surface with red, irritated outer margins and pale scaly centers.

Although the temptation to scratch these sometimes itchy skin infections is often irresistible, to do so merely increases the possibility of spreading the fungi on to new areas of the body, including the fingernails.

Fungal infections of the beard ("barber's itch" or Tinea barbae): Fungal infections of the beard are much less common today than they were in the past, although they still occur. The fungi that cause Tinea barbae infect beard hairs, producing soft swelling inflammation, ringwormlike sores, and small pustules within the hair follicles. In time, the hairs become dull and brittle and eventually shed or simply break off with the possibility of permanent loss.

The name barber's itch originated because this ailment was spread by barbers from one customer to another via brushes and razors. Farmers were particularly affected because their livestock served as a reservoir for the tiny fungal plants.

Today, infection still occurs among farmers, but the ailment is in no way limited to them. Anyone can contract this disease, and household pets frequently take the place of livestock as a potential source of infection.

Fungal infections of the nails (Tinea unguium): When fingernails or toenails are infected with fungi, the disease is called Tinea unguium. Germinating at the edge of the nail and extending under the nail borders, the fungi that cause this infection will progressively occupy the entire nail bed. At any time in the early course of this illness, the fungi can become static with only minor nail change resulting. However, with increased growth and deep-seated infection, nail degeneration becomes apparent.

Initially, only lateral opacity is noted but, with time, the entire nail may lose luster, thicken, and distort. Progressive changes may continue until the entire nail, lifted up and separated from the underlying nail plate, becomes a crumbling sheet of discolored protein, leaving a naked nail bed and thousands of fungi ready and able to infect again. Women are particularly affected.

Fungal infections of the feet ("athlete's foot," Tinea pedis): The fungi that cause athlete's foot, also known as Tinea pedis, thrive on the damp, dusky privacy provided by shoes, socks, and sweaty feet. They produce symptoms consisting chiefly of scaling, itching, odor, and, more severely, painful open cuts that frequently develop behind the little toe. This is not to say the other toes will be spared, however. Athlete's foot fungi will grow anywhere a supportive environment can be found and, if given the chance, will spread to the under surface of the toes and possibly to the bottom of the foot as well.

Although many studies have been made regarding the

acquisition of Tinea pedis, inconclusive evidence has been obtained thus far. For example, it is difficult to discover fungi growing in gymnasiums, showers, ponds, or locker rooms, areas traditionally considered to be hideouts for the opportunistic plants. Equally perplexing is the fact that transmission from individual to individual seems unlikely since direct contact with the toes rarely produces infection even in the face of poor hygiene.

Amid this uncertainty, several pertinent facts do arise. First, athlete's foot is an ailment of certain adult men who seemingly have an increased susceptibility that cannot be readily explained. Second, since athlete's foot is virtually unknown among people who go barefoot, apparently shoes increase the susceptibility factor by retaining moisture, promoting warmth, and creating darkness.

Fungal infections of the groin ("jock itch," Tinea cruris): Tinea cruris is the fungal infection of the groin. It usually begins as a small red patch in the skin folds of the upper leg, then spreads to the inner surface of the thighs and possibly on to the genital and anal skin. New growth expands with a well-delineated margin, consisting of small blisters or pimples that outline the older inner patches that usually turn from red to reddish brown. Itching is a prominent feature.

Fungal infections of the upper torso (Tinea versicolor): Tinea versicolor is a fungal infection of changing color, so aptly expressed in its name and demonstrated by the brown, beige, and white hues taken on by individual fungal patches as they grow on the chest, shoulders, and back. Apparently, sun exposure enhances the intensity of color in some patches, while others seemingly become lighter in contrast to normal skin tanning. The lesions will measure up to one inch in diameter and have no prominent symptoms other than looking unsightly and giving the affected area a spotted appearance.

What is Candida?
Candida is a specific fungus that causes infections that frequently resemble the Tineas in appearance and symptoms. Unfortunately, Candida infections do not respond to

the OTC antifungal medications and must be treated with prescription drugs.

Candida infections occur in the groin, arm pits, under the breasts, and in the corners of the mouth. Involvement of the hands and nails is occasionally noted, especially in adults who frequently immerse their hands in soapy water.

Because Candida infections are associated with a white creamy discharge, distinction from the Tineas is possible. This discharge, in conjunction with sore, itchy, red fungal patches, may be noted in the corners of the mouth or in the body skin folds of the groin, arm pits, breasts, and thighs. It commonly occurs in women around the vagina and genitals, especially during pregnancy.

If Candida is suspected, the doctor must be consulted.

What can be done to treat superficial fungal infections?

The choice of treatment depends on the severity of the infection. Nonprescription drugs usually contain one or more of the following medications:

Benzoic and salicylic acid ointment (Whitfield's ointment): Whitfield's ointment combines the antifungal activities of benzoic acid with the loosening, peeling action that salicylic acid has on the skin. As the infected or dead skin peels away, benzoic acid attacks the underlying fungi. The ointment is used primarily for athlete's foot and occasionally for fungal scalp infections. Local irritation may result following application.

Selenium sulfide: Selenium sulfide is found in several dandruff shampoos. Not only is it effective in controlling dandruff, its usefulness extends to the treatment of Tinea versicolor as well. Slight skin irritation may occur at the site of application, but this is rare.

Tolnaftate: Considered to be the most effective OTC antifungal agent, tolnaftate can be used against all the superficial fungi except Candida. Generally, infections of the nails, hands, and feet are slow to respond, and scalp infections may fail to respond at all. When this occurs, oral medication obtained by prescription is necessary. With thickened scaly sores, tolnaftate should be applied after 10 percent salicylic acid has been used to loosen the dead matted skin. Toxic effects of this drug are virtually nonexistent.

Triacetin: Triacetin has a limited antifungal activity due to the slow release of acetic acid that results when this compound decomposes. Effectiveness is questionable.

Undecylenic acid and zinc: Undecylenic acid alone or in combination with zinc also has limited antifungal activity. It has a moderately beneficial effect in the treatment of athlete's foot, but infections usually persist. The zinc found in these preparations helps to reduce inflammation.

RECOMMENDED TREATMENT
Superficial fungal infections, although in no way life threatening, are unsightly and annoying because of the burning, tenderness, and extreme itching they produce. Treatment varies depending on the site and extent of infection and is usually quite prolonged because of the resistant nature of the fungal organisms.

Tolnaftate is the best therapeutic agent available over the counter and, since it is effective against the great majority of skin fungi, it can be used with the confidence that totally resistant organisms are few in number. Treatment should begin as soon as the infection is discovered, because the longer the delay in therapy, the more difficult the infection is to treat.

COMMENTS AND CAUTIONS
Treatment of superficial fungal infections with OTC topical medications may take weeks or months to be effective. Even after months of therapy, infection can persist, in which case prescription drugs must be used. At times, even prescription drugs fail to cure deep-seated fungal disease, but generally good results will follow prolonged use. If a fungal infection fails to respond to self-medication with OTC products, see your doctor.

FUNGICIDES

Boldface: Recommended

Aftate, liquid, powder, gel

tolnaftate 1%

Bevill's, lotion

salicylic acid
alcohol 68%
ether 8%
methyl salicylate 1%

Blis-To-Sol, gel

undecylenic acid 5%

Blis-To-Sol, liquid

undecylenic acid 50 mg/1 g
salicylic acid 90 mg/1 g

Blis-To-Sol, aerosol powder

zinc stearate 10 mg/1 g
salicylic acid 10 mg/1 g
benzoic acid 10 mg/1 g

Blis-To-Sol, powder

zinc stearate 10 mg/1 g
salicylic acid 19 mg/1 g
benzoic acid 19 mg/1 g

Campho-Phenique, liquid

phenol 4.75%
camphor 10.86%

Campho-Phenique, powder

phenol 2%
camphor 4.38%

Daliderm, powder

zinc undecylenate
sodium propionate
salicylic acid
methylbenzethonium chloride
corn starch
magnesium carbonate
boric acid
bentonite
zinc oxide
talc
aromatic oils

Desenex, ointment

zinc undecylenate 20%
undecylenic acid 5%

Desenex, powder, aerosol

zinc undecylenate 20%
undecylenic acid 2%

Desenex, soap	undecylenic acid 2%
Desenex, liquid	undecylenic acid 10% isopropyl alchhol propylene glycol triethanolamine
Deso-Creme	zinc undecylenate 20% caprylic acid 5% sodium propionate 2%
Enzactin, cream	triacetin 250 mg
Enzactin, spray	triacetin 15%
Enzactin, powder	triacetin 33.3%
Fungacetin, liquid	triacetin 30%
Fungacetin, ointment	triacetin 25%
Fungacetin, powder	triacetin 33.3%
Jim Wade Deodorant Foot Powder	8-hydroxyquinoline 0.01% aluminum sulfate 15% menthol 1% corn starch boric acid talc
Jim Wade Foot Medicine	salicylic acid sucrose octaacetate acetone
NP 27, aerosol powder	zinc undecylenate salicylic acid dichlorophene
NP 27, cream	8-hydroxyquinoline sulfate salicylic acid benzoic acid propylparaben methylparaben

NP 27, liquid

salicylic acid
isopropyl alcohol
benzoic acid
propylparaben
benzyl alcohol
chlorothymol

NP 27, powder

salicylic acid
benzoic acid
eucalyptol
menthol

Podiaspray

undecylenic acid
salicylic acid
cetyltrimethylammonium bromide
chloroxylenol
aromatic base

Quinsana, foot
powder

zinc undecylenate 20%
undecylenic acid 2%

Rid-Itch, cream

zinc undecylenate 20%
undecylenic acid 5%
2–(2–35 hoxyethoxy) ethanol
emulsion base

Rid-Itch, liquid

salicylic acid 7%
boric acid 5%
benzoic acid 2%
resorcinol 1%
chlorothymol 1%
alcohol
glycerin

Salicresen, liquid

salicylic acid 2%
acetone 10%
benzoic acid 2%
secondary amyltricresols 0.1%
o-hydroxyphenylmercuric chloride 0.1%
alcohol

Solvex, ointment

salicylic acid
thymol
benzoic acid

Solvex, powder

8-hydroxyquinoline sulfate
colloidal sulfur
salicylic acid
chlorothymol

Solvex, spray

undecylenic acid
dichlorophene
chlorothymol
benzocaine
propylene glycol
alcohol

Sopronol, liquid

sodium propionate 12.3%
sodium caprylate 10%

Sopronol, ointment

sodium propionate 12.3%
sodium caprylate 10%
zinc caprylate 5%

Sopronol, powder

sodium propionate 5%
sodium caprylate 10%
zinc propionate 5%

Tinactin, liquid

tolnaftate 1%
polyethylene glycol 400
butylated hydroxytoluene

Tinactin, cream

tolnaftate 1%
polyethylene glycol 400
propylene glycol
butylated hydroxytoluene
titanium dioxide

Tinactin, powder

tolnaftate 1%
corn starch
talc

Tinactin, aerosol
powder

tolnaftate 1%
talc
butylated hydroxytoluene
propellants

Ting, cream

zinc stearate
benzoic acid
boric acid
zinc oxide
alcohol

Ting, powder

zinc stearate
benzoic acid
boric acid
zinc oxide

Verdefam, cream

propionic acid 3%
undecylenic acid 2%
sodium propionate 1%
sodium caprylate 1%
copper undecylenate 0.5%
salicylic acid 3%

Verdefam, solution

undecylenic acid 5%
propionic acid 3%
sodium propionate 2%
sodium caprylate 2%
copper undecylenate 0.5%
salicylic acid 5%

Zea SORB, powder

microporous cellulose 45%
p-chloro-m xylenol 0.5%
aluminum dehydroxy allantoinate 0.2%

22. Headache

Where does headache pain originate?
Contrary to what one would ordinarily think, headache pain does not originate in the brain. In fact, actual brain tissue is insensitive to pain because it has no pain fibers. Where, then, does headache pain come from?

Although the brain, itself, cannot cause pain, some of the fibrous tissue that covers the brain can. And the blood vessels that are found within the fibrous covering (meninges) are also pain sensitive. But these are not the only structures that elicit pain. The specialized parts of the head, the eyes, ears, nose, and sinuses, are responsible for some headache pain, while the scalp, head and neck muscles, and the cranial nerves are the sites of others.

Pain arises when blood vessels, nerves, and meninges are stretched, pressurized, or compressed and when spasms develop in the head and neck muscles.

Why, then, can something like a brain tumor produce a constant headache?
With a little thought, the answer becomes obvious. Although the tumor might grow deep within the brain substance, in time, it will exert pressure or stretch those structures within the head that are pain sensitive—arteries, veins, nerves, meninges—and then produce pain that is perceived as a constant, progressively worsening headache.

What are other specific causes for headaches?
Cluster headaches: Occurring mostly in men, cluster headaches are very characteristic. They usually affect one

side of the face, particularly around the eyes, and begin two to three hours after falling asleep. The pain, which is usually extreme, is associated with tearing, nasal congestion, or a runny nose. Swelling and reddening of the painful area might also develop.

Generally, cluster headaches will occur every night for weeks to months, then not recur for years, thus the name "cluster headaches." In several ways they are similar to migraine headaches and, consequently, are thought to be caused by blood vessels in the head.

Hypertensive (high blood pressure) headaches: Principally noted in the morning and affecting the top and back of the head, hypertensive headaches are caused by intracranial blood vessels. As the pressure within these vessels increases, their walls are stretched, and headache pain results. Slight swelling of the brain, due to the higher blood pressure, may also pull or stretch the meninges and add to the pain.

Migraine headaches: Like cluster headaches, migraine headaches are very distinctive. Usually they begin early in life, frequently before adolescence. And, they often affect several members of the same family.

Before an attack begins, some type of visual or hearing disturbance is noted, possibly blind spots before the eyes or ringing in the ears. Then the pain commences.

Characteristically located on one side of the head, migraine headache pain starts with a throbbing, then progresses to an intense, constant ache. Nausea and vomiting may occur.

These headaches are caused by arteries within the brain. First they narrow, then they widen, leading to the distressing pain of migraines.

Tension headaches: These are the common headaches. They are the result of tension or spasms in the muscles of the head and neck and usually occur later in the day. Generally, the pain begins at the base of the skull and projects to the side of the head. One or both sides may be affected.

Sinus headaches: As infected sinuses fill during the night, the sensitive sinus lining becomes pressurized, and sinus headache pain gradually develops. Consequently, the pain is most intense in the morning upon awakening. During the day when an erect stature is maintained and the sinuses have a chance to drain, the pain subsides. Nasal sprays and decongestants will help to relieve sinus headache pain. See Chapter 7, "Colds and Flus" (pages 59-62, 64-65, 66).

The upper face and forehead are the major sites of sinus headache pain.

Ocular (eye) headaches: Eye headaches have two main causes. First, they may occur following prolonged use of the eyes for reading or other close work. In this case, the muscles of the eyes are responsible for the pain.

Secondly, ocular headaches may be caused by diseases within the eye, mainly, infections or glaucoma (a disease of increased ocular pressure).

Usually eye headaches produce pain about the eye, but discomfort may project deeper into the head or up along the forehead.

Traumatic headaches: Headaches that result from injury to the head are called traumatic headaches. They can take several forms.

Immediately after a head injury, pain may be noted because the brain has been rapidly displaced in one direction, then the other, with resultant stretching of vessels and meninges. Scalp and muscular nerves may also be bruised, contributing to the pain. But these headaches are short-lived and usually of no real consequence.

Far more serious problems occasionally develop following head injury and usually are associated with some form of headache.

If blood vessels are torn in the course of an injury, bleeding will occur over the surface of the brain. When this happens, headaches slowly develop and are associated with a variety of other symptoms, which include visual disturbances, personality changes, dizziness, drowsiness, muscular weakness, and possibly even coma. This condition, known as a subdural hematoma (blood under the meninges), develops over a period of weeks to months and can prove to be fatal if medical treatment is delayed.

Brain tumor headaches: As previously mentioned, brain tumors will give rise to headaches, but are low on the list of causes. Unfortunately, the headaches that are caused by brain tumors are almost totally indistinct. They may come and go several times in one day or may last for several days. They can be located anywhere in the head, primarily relating to the position of the tumor. And, they may be associated with many other symptoms. Headaches caused by brain tumors tend to become progressively more frequent and more severe as the tumor enlarges.

Headaches of meningitis: Meningitis, which is an inflammation of the meninges, causes a distinctive type of headache that is rapid in onset, generalized, constant, and severe. The most characteristic quality of these headaches is the increase in pain that is noted when the head is tilted forward. Frequently, the pain is so intense, the chin cannot be brought in contact with the chest. Nausea and vomiting may be present.

It is thought that the pain of meningial headaches is due to irritation of the nerves in the meninges.

RECOMMENDED TREATMENT

Since common headaches are caused by tension and spasms of the muscles of the head and neck, relaxation is important and can be accomplished in several ways. Gentle massage will aid tense, spastic muscles and provide relief. Heat applied to the back of the head and neck will accomplish the same goal. A short period of rest or a hot shower should also help. Relaxation is the key.

Where pain is annoying and relaxation cannot be achieved, aspirin or acetaminophen will work wonders. Use these drugs discriminately.

Refer to Chapter 1, on "Aches and Pains" (pages 5-6) for cautions and side effects.

COMMENTS AND CAUTIONS

The only headaches that should be self-medicated are common headaches. All others should be evaluated by a doctor. If you note that your headaches are similar to migraines, sinus headaches, or any of the other headaches described in this chapter, go to your personal physician for a thorough examination. Urgency is especially important when the headaches are associated with the signs of meningitis, subdural hematoma or high blood pressure. All long-standing headaches, regardless of their nature, require professional evaluation, too.

MILD PAIN RELIEVERS

For a listing of these medications, please turn to Chapter 1, "Aches and Pains" (pages 6-14).

23. Hemorrhoids

What, exactly, are hemorrhoids?
Hemorrhoids are varicose veins of the rectum and anus.

How are varicose veins different from ordinary veins?
Normal veins are able to maintain their natural tubular shape, but varicose veins balloon into odd sizes and shapes because their walls are weak and worn out.

What causes rectal varicose veins and hemorrhoids?
Many different explanations for rectal varicose veins and hemorrhoids have been advanced through the years, but the precise reason for their occurrence is evasive. Perhaps they occur because, unlike our primitive animal ancestors, we stand erect and, in doing so, allow blood to gravitate to the lower parts of our bodies, where it engorges and dilates weaker veins in the legs, rectum, and anus. No doubt, heredity plays some role, since individuals whose parents have hemorrhoids are likely to develop them also.

More specific causes exist, too. For example, anything that applies pressure to rectal veins will obstruct the flow of blood and lead to varicosities and hemorrhoids. Pressure might arise from the weight of a developing baby during a pregnancy, from straining to move the bowels during periods of constipation or from attempting to urinate with prostatic enlargement. Regardless of the specific cause, it is pressure in rectal veins that produces the stretching and ballooning that leads to hemorrhoids.

Are there different types of hemorrhoids?
Basically there are two types of hemorrhoids and their differences mainly depend on their locations. Internal hem-

orrhoids, those that develop within the rectum, are caused by engorgement and enlargement of the internal rectal veins. External hemorrhoids arise from varicose veins of the external rectal network and extend around the outside of the anus just under the skin.

What do hemorrhoids look like?
This also depends on their location. Small internal hemorrhoids, those located within the rectum, are usually little red purple clumps that protrude from the rectal wall. If they enlarge, they may actually droop lower in the rectum or extend out of the anus, suspended by small thin stalks. External hemorrhoids basically have the same red purple color, but they are found along the rim of the anus, where they either protrude under the anal skin or dangle in grapelike clusters from the anal surface.

Who suffers from hemorrhoids?
About 35 percent of the population suffers from hemorrhoids. Of these 75 million people, the great majority are between twenty-five and fifty-five years of age. Men and women are equally affected.

Are serious medical problems ever associated with hemorrhoids?
Yes, they are. Since tumors of the rectum, bladder, prostate, and uterus can all create pressure in rectal veins, they can also produce hemorrhoids. Because cirrhosis of the liver can cause a backup of blood in all intestinal veins, including the rectal veins, this disease is occasionally associated with hemorrhoids too. Fortunately, most cases of hemorrhoids result from far less significant problems, but the more serious illnesses must always be kept in mind whenever hemorrhoids form.

What are the complications of hemorrhoids?
There are three major complications of hemorrhoids.

Prolapse: As mentioned before, hemorrhoids may actually enlarge enough to hang from the anus or out of the rectum. When this happens, they are called prolapsed hemorrhoids.

Thrombosis: Because blood often stagnates in varicose veins, clots sometimes develop and partially, or completely, interrupt blood flow. Thrombosis is the term that applies to plugged blood vessels and describes those hemorrhoids (thrombosed hemorrhoids) that contain occlusive blood clots.

Irritation and infection: Hemorrhoids usually become irritated and, possibly, ulcerated as fecal material passes over them and bruises them during bowel movements. As the irritation and ulceration become contaminated by bacteria, infection may result.

Do hemorrhoids always produce symptoms?

Initially, when hemorrhoids are just forming, there may be no indication of their presence; however, as they enlarge, symptoms will develop.

Usually the first sign is minor bleeding. Blood may be noted on toilet tissue, underwear, or passed stools. With continued enlargement, irritation results and is soon followed by itching and burning. Pain may also occur if the hemorrhoids become thrombosed.

Thus, the major symptoms of hemorrhoids are itching, burning, and pain, but these telltale signs do not appear until the hemorrhoids enlarge significantly.

Can hemorrhoids be confused with other ailments?

Yes, they can. The itching, burning, and pain that occurs with hemorrhoids may also arise with other medical problems. Small cracks or fissures occasionally develop in the skin around the anus and have the same signs and symptoms as hemorrhoids. Anal discomfort is common to a condition known as cryptitis, which is irritation and enlargement of the anal valves. And, intestinal parasites (pin worms) frequently cause itching around the rectal outlet, which might be misinterpreted as hemorrhoid irritations.

More serious problems, like tumors, abscesses, and abnormal intestinal passages called fistulas, may also produce rectal swelling, pain, and bleeding which might also be confused with hemorrhoids. As mentioned before, these conditions sometimes even cause hemorrhoids.

What constitutes proper treatment of hemorrhoids?
The treatment of simple, uncomplicated hemorrhoids merely requires conservative control of symptoms like itching, swelling, and minor pain. Large prolapsed or thrombosed hemorrhoids are more properly treated by special medical and surgical techniques that necessitate professional assistance.

Eliminating the mild annoying symptoms of hemorrhoids may be accomplished by conforming to the following suggestions:

1. Eat bulky foods, leafy vegetables, fruits, and grains, which will help regulate bowel movements and keep stools soft. The use of a stool softener is advisable when dry, hard stools are troublesome. Laxatives may also be used for constipation in order to avoid straining at the stool.
2. Don't lift heavy weights or perform other activities that increase pressure in the abdomen.
3. Warm-water soaks or sitting baths should be initiated when discomfort occurs.
4. Following a bowel movement, pat yourself clean with a damp washcloth. Avoid excessive wiping with bathroom tissues.

Are there any over-the-counter products for hemorrhoid sufferers?
There is a large variety of hemorrhoid products available over the counter. They consist of anesthetics, antiseptics, astringents, and substances that cause blood vessels to constrict (vasoconstrictors) or promote wound healing (vitamins and skin respiratory factors). Here are the most common kinds of medications:

Anesthetics: Local anesthetics will reduce the superficial pain, itching, and burning of hemorrhoids if they are applied in sufficient quantities. OTC products contain benzocaine, diperodon, pramoxine, dibucaine, and tetracaine. These products may cause allergic reactions in susceptible individuals.

Antiseptics: Antiseptics are commonly used to clean

wounds and sores. By reducing the number of bacteria present around irritated tissues, they help to prevent infections. However, in view of the tremendous number of bacteria in the intestines and the low concentration of antiseptics in over-the-counter preparations, these substances have little effect on hemorrhoids.

Astringents: Alcohol, bismuth salts, hamamelis water, and zinc oxide are the astringents found in hemorrhoid products. They help to relieve swelling and inflammation of the hemorrhoids through an effect on the walls of small blood vessels.

Vasoconstrictors: Vasoconstrictors also produce an effect on the walls of small blood vessels. Through an action on the microscopic muscles that are present in arteries, vasoconstrictors cause these blood vessels to narrow. However, veins respond very poorly, and dilated veins are the basic problem common to all hemorrhoids.

Wound healers: Some substances found in hemorrhoid preparations (balsam of Peru, skin respiratory factor from shark liver oil and yeast, plus vitamins A and D) are supposed to promote wound healing. Of this group, skin respiratory factor has been shown to stimulate cell growth that is needed for wound repair.

RECOMMENDED TREATMENT
Products that contain benzocaine in 20 percent solution will relieve the itching and burning of irritated internal and external hemorrhoids. These products will also control similar symptoms caused by other minor anal and rectal disorders. For minor internal hemorrhoids, products that contain astringents and wound-healing skin respiratory factor should relieve minor swelling and irritation. If minor pain becomes troublesome, a minor pain reliever such as aspirin will prove helpful.

COMMENTS AND CAUTIONS
Hemorrhoids are the most common cause of rectal bleeding. If you notice fresh red blood on toilet paper, hem-

orrhoids are likely present. Other forms of rectal bleeding, far more serious than hemorrhoids, also exist and must be treated immediately by a doctor. When the blood you notice is mixed in with your stool or imparts a dark red brown, or even black, color to your stool, make an appointment with your doctor; you have something more than simple hemorrhoids.

HEMORRHOIDAL MEDICATIONS

Boldface: Recommended

A-Caine, ointment	benzocaine 2% zinc oxide 5% pyrilamine maleate 0.1% phenylephrine 0.255% diperodon hydrochloride 0.25% carbonate 0.2%
Americaine, **ointment**	benzocaine 20% benzethonium chloride 0.1% polyethylene glycol base
Americaine, suppository	benzocaine 280 mg benzethonium chloride 0.1% polyethylene glycol base
Anusol ointment, suppository	zinc oxide 11% bismuth subgallate 2.5% balsam of Peru 1.8% bismuth resorcinol compound 1.75% benzyl benzoate 1.2% vegetable oil base
Aphco, ointment, suppository	benzocaine zinc oxide boric acid balsam of Peru bismuth salts
BiCozene, cream	benzocaine 6% resorcinol 1.67% cream base

Blue-Gray, suppository	benzocaine zinc oxide boric acid bismuth subgallate bismuth resorcinol compound balsam of Peru
Calmol 4, suppository	zinc oxide bismuth subgallate balsam of Peru cod liver oil cocoa butter base
Diothane, ointment	diperodon 1% benzoxyquine 0.1% propylene glycol sorbital sesquioleate
Eudicane, suppository	benzocaine 130 mg zinc oxide 260 mg bismuth subgallate 64.8 mg balsam of Peru 64.8 mg 8-hydroxyquinoline sulfate 16.2 mg ephedrine sulfate 4.05 mg
Gentz Wipes, medical pad	hamamelis water 50% pramoxine hydrochloride 1% cetylpyridinium chloride 0.5% aluminum chlorhydroxyallantoinate 0.2% propylene glycol 0.10%
Hazel Balm, aerosol	hamamelis water 79.9% lanolin derivative 20% benzethonium chloride 0.1%
Hemor-Rid, ointment	diperodon hydrochloride 0.25% zinc oxide 5% pyrilamine maleate 0.1% phenylephrine hydrochloride 0.25% bismuth subcarbonate 0.2% cod liver oil petrolatum
Lanacane, cream	benzocaine phenylmercuric acetate 0.02% chlorothymol resorcinol water base

Mamol, ointment

bismuth subnitrate 40%

Manzan, ointment

benzocaine 1%
tannic acid 0.5%
phenol 0.5%
allantoin 0.5%
menthol 0.2%
ephedrine hydrochloride 0.2%

Manzan Stainless,
ointment

benzocaine 1%
zinc oxide 10%
phenol 0.5%
allantoin 0.5%
ephedrine hydrochloride 0.2%

Manzan,
suppositories

benzocaine 1%
zinc oxide 96%
phenol 0.5%
menthol 0.2%
allantoin 0.2%
phenylpropanolamine hydrochloride 0.2%

Mediconet, medical
pad

hamamelis water 50%
glycerin 10%
lanolin 0.5%
methylparaben 0.15%
benzalkonium chloride 0.02%

Nupercainal,
ointment

dibucaine 1%
acetone sodium bisulfite 0.5%

Nupercainal,
suppositories

dibucaine 2.5 mg
zinc oxide
acetone sodium bisulfite 0.05%
bismuth subgallate
cocoa butter

Pazo, ointment

benzocaine 0.8%
zinc oxide 4%
camphor 2.18%
ephedrine sulfate 0.2%
eucalyptus oil 0.25%
lanolin 0.05%
petrolatum

Pazo, suppositories

benzocaine 0.8%
zinc oxide 4%
camphor 2.18%
ephedrine sulfate 0.2%
eucalyptus oil 0.25%
vegetable oil

PNS, suppositories

tetracaine hydrochloride 10 mg
bismuth subcarbonate 100 mg
phenylephrine hydrochloride 5 mg
tyloxapol 25 mg

**Preparation H,
ointment,
suppository**

shark liver oil 3%
phenylmercuric nitrate 0.01%
skin respiratory factor 2000 units
(from live yeast cell derivative)

Proctodon, cream

diperodon hydrochloride 1%

Proctofoam, foam

pramoxine hydrochloride 1%
mineral oil

Rantex, medical pad

hamamelis water 50%
alcohol 7%
benzalkonium chloride
methylparaben
lanolin

Rectal Medicone,
suppository

benzocaine 130 mg
zinc oxide 195 mg
balsam of Peru 65 mg
8-hydroxyquinoline sulfate 16.25 mg
menthol 9.3 mg
cocoa butter
vegetable oil
petroleum oil

Rectal Medicone,
Unguent, ointment

benzocaine 20 mg
zinc oxide 100 mg
balsam of Peru 12.5 mg
8-hydroxyquinoline sulfate 5 mg
menthol 5 mg
petrolatum
lanolin

Tanicaine, ointment

phenacaine hydrochloride 325 mg/30 ml
zinc oxide 5.2 g/30 ml
tannic acid 1.6 g/30 ml
camphor 455 mg/30 ml
phenol 390/30 ml
menthol 130 mg/30 ml
atropine 16.25 mg/30 ml

Tanicaine,
suppositories

phenacaine hydrochloride 22 mg
zinc oxide 390 mg
tannic acid 110 mg
phenol 13 mg
atropine 1 mg

Tucks, cream,
ointment

hamamelis water 50%
lanolin
petrolatum

Tucks, pads

hamamelis water 50%
glycerin 10%
methylparaben 0.1%
benzalkonium chloride 0.003%

Vaseline Hemorr-
Aid, ointment

petrolatum 100%

Wyanoid, ointment

benzocaine 2%
zinc oxide 5%
boric acid 18%
balsam of Peru 1%
ephedrine sulfate 0.1%
castor oil
petrolatum

Wyanoid,
suppositories

zinc oxide 176 mg
boric acid 543 mg
bismuth subcarbonate 146 mg
bismuth oxiodide 30 mg
balsam of Peru 30 mg
belladonna extract 15 mg
ephedrine sulfate 3 mg
cocoa butter

24. Insect Bites and Stings

What insects commonly bite humans?
Quite a few. Here is a list of the most prevalent.

Bedbugs: Bedbugs are very small creatures that bite into the skin with one set of jaws, then swallow blood from the wound through an inner sucker. Their bite may go completely unnoticed or may swell, itch, and become red.

Caterpillars: Although these small furry creepers don't bite, they occasionally cause bitelike reactions. The swelling, itching, pain, and blister formation that results after handling a caterpillar may also follow contact with caterpillar fuzz or even cocoons. The reaction is caused by toxins released from the surface of the insect.

Centipedes: Causing mild skin irritation to extensive death of body tissues and pain, centipedes are unpredictable pests. Occasionally, severe reactions result from the bite of tropical species, and generalized poisoning is noted. Centipede bites are more common in the southern and western parts of the United States.

Chiggers, red bugs: The small red larvae (immature forms) of the chigger cause extreme itching and raised, red skin patches when they attack and bite into the skin. The larvae, themselves, are red and can occasionally be seen in the center of the sore, sucking blood.

Fleas: These bloodsuckers can easily be seen on the covered or hairy parts of the body because of their size and jumping abilities. Like the other biting insects described above, the flea bores through the skin, then feasts on the victim's blood. Flea bites tend to be multiple and grouped together; they itch intensely.

Flies: Several different types of flies bite humans, and although the actual bite is painful, serious side effects are rare.

Lice: Lice are crablike parasites that survive on blood. They prefer the body parts and usually can be found on the head, in the arm pits, and around the groin, where they live and lay eggs. Their bites produce round, red, raised skin sores.

Mosquitos: These long-nosed insects are all too well known. Although attacking humans in the evening is the rule, these menacing little pests will bite any time. They gnaw through the skin, then extend their long hollow suckers into the wound in search of blood. Generally, only minor swelling and itching will result from the bite.

Ticks: The skin irritation that develops following a tick bite is usually insignificant, that is, if the tick's head and mouth are removed with the body of the animal. When the mouth parts are left in place, a firm, itchy nodule may develop. Ticks will attach to the skin and suck blood until their bodies are markedly enlarged and distended. They will remain firmly fixed to the body for several days, if they are not removed.

One very important complication of tick bites is tick paralysis. Infrequently, while a tick is attached to the skin and sucking blood, a mild paralysis, muscle weakness, loss of coordination, and poor reflexes will occur. The precise cause of this paralysis is unknown, but it will go away within a few days if the offending tick or ticks are removed. Failure to locate and completely detach the responsible tick will result in worse paralysis and possibly even death.

Spiders: Spider bites may produce simple, local skin soreness or extreme general poisoning and even death. The degree of illness relates to the type of spider, the amount of venom released with the bite, and the susceptibility of the victim (children and elderly adults are most susceptible). Approximately fifty deaths occur each year in the United States from spider bites.

With poison bites, cramping pain begins in about thirty minutes and spreads from the bite site to various parts of the body. Breathing may eventually become difficult. Nausea, vomiting, headaches, twitching, and paralysis may also occur. If the spider bite has gone unnoticed, the exact cause for such extreme illness may be difficult to pinpoint.

What insects commonly sting humans?
The most common are ants, bees, and wasps.

Ants can bite and sting at the same time. They use their jaws to bite and attach to their victims, then they sting the bitten area with venom released from their abdomen. The results of all this biting and stinging are itching, redness, and pimple formation with pus.

Bees and wasps produce local pain, swelling, and redness when they jab their stinger into the skin and inject poison through their hollow stinger into the wound. Since wasps have barbless stingers, they can attack their victim over and over again until their store of venom is depleted. Bees that have a barb on the end of their stinger, can only assault their prey once, because the stinger stays in the skin and with it remain the poison glands. These bees subsequently die.

What are the possible complications of insect bites and stings?
There are many possible complications of insect bites and stings. Some are minor and easily treated; others are catastrophic and actually require national or international attention. For example, mosquitos transmit malaria by feasting on the blood of infected birds and reptiles, then biting man. They are also capable of spreading encephalitis (an inflammation of the brain) and yellow fever (the disease that almost prevented the building of the Panama Canal). Typhus fever is spread by lice. Rocky Mountain spotted fever is transmitted by the bite of a tick. Flea bites aided the spread of the notorious plague, the disease that devastated the world many years ago. Other less serious complications of insect bites and stings include allergic reactions and infections that occur on an individual basis.

How do bites and stings cause allergic reactions?
The saliva of the biting insects and the venom of the stinging insects produce an exaggerated response in some people.

After a bite or sting, antibodies (small proteins which attack foreign substances) are produced by the body. Normally, these antibodies neutralize the toxins of the insect; but in sensitized people, they function improperly and cause additional problems, which include severe local irritation at the site of the bite or sting, hives, vomiting, fainting, breathing difficulty, shock, and sometimes death.

How do bites and stings cause infections?
Insects may cause infections by introducing bacteria, viruses, or other small organisms into the wounds they produce when they bite or sting. In this manner, malaria, yellow fever, and other specific diseases previously mentioned are started and spread.

Bacteria, which are always present on the skin, may find a bite or sting ideal for their growth and reproduction. Entering the small wound produced by the insect, they feed on the blood and dying tissues, producing additional injury themselves. Ultimately, pustules or abscesses may form and, in extreme cases, general sickness can ensure. Scratching or rubbing insect bites and stings helps to introduce germs into these sores.

What is scabies?
Scabies is a skin infection characterized by itching, redness, and encrusted infected sores. The disease is caused by a mite that burrows into the skin, then reproduces and lays eggs in the small skin trenches. When the eggs hatch, the young mites continue to burrow and reproduce. The burrows, small black lines in the skin, can usually be seen between the fingers, on the wrists, in the skin folds of the arm pits, and around the genitals. Frequently, the small, white, shiny mite can be seen at one end of the burrow mark. Although the mite sores can be self-treated, additional measures must be taken to get rid of the mites. See your doctor.

What can be done for insect bites and stings?
Following an insect bite or sting, several measures may be taken to reduce the local reaction, help prevent infection, and minimize the possibility of serious allergic complica-

tions. These measures include first aid, the use of skin lotions and creams, oral medications, and emergency medications.

First aid: Stings and bites should be washed with cold water and soap as soon as possible. Then, an antiseptic and ice should be applied to the wound. If the sting is from a bee and the stinger is left within the skin, it should be removed immediately. Since a small venom pouch is attached to the stinger, removal should be gentle and performed with a light scratching motion of a fingernail or tweezer. The venom sac should never be squeezed because more poison will be injected into the wound.

When ticks are removed from the body, the head must also be withdrawn from the skin. Frequently, touching the tick with a hot match head or a piece of ice will cause the nasty animal to release its sucking grip, and the entire tick, head and all, can easily be removed. Again, an antiseptic should be applied to the wound following a thorough washing.

Skin lotions and creams: The itching and irritation caused by biting and stinging insects can be reduced by the application of an appropriate lotion, ointment, or cream. Such products include astringents (alcohol, calamine, zinc oxide), which supposedly draw toxins from the bite or sting; antibacterial medications (alcohol, benzethonium chloride), which kill germs; antihistamines (methapyrilene, tripelennamine), which relieve itching and swelling; local anesthetics (benzocaine, phenol), which reduce pain and possibly relieve itching; and numerous other ingredients.

Oral medications: These consist primarily of antihistamines and can be very effective in reducing swelling, relieving itch, and preventing allergic complications caused by the release of histamine in the body. These medications should be taken immediately after a bite or sting because they will take approximately thirty minutes to be effective.

Emergency medications: Emergency medications such as epinephrine, isoproterenol, steroids, and certain antihistamines are available by prescription only and can be found in kit form. These products are intended for those people who demonstrate severe allergic reactions to insect bites and stings and should be used only by people who have been instructed in their proper administration.

Why does the treatment vary?
The severity of the reaction to a bite or sting determines which treatment should be used. First aid measures should always be applied in order to reduce the possibility of infection and also to limit the extent of the reaction as much as possible. When local irritation is annoying because of itching or soreness, a topical lotion or cream can be used to diminish the discomfort. If a person is sensitive to the bite or sting of different insects, an oral antihistamine should be taken immediately following the attack. Hopefully, this will prevent any excessive reaction. Finally, emergency treatment is needed only when someone has an extreme sensitivity and faces the possibility of shock or death following a bite or sting. Generally, we each know what category we fall into and what method of treatment is best for us.

RECOMMENDED TREATMENT

I prefer creams of lotions rather than ointments. Generally, the local anesthetics, such as benzocaine, that are used in these preparations are present in insufficient quantities to adequately penetrate the skin. Similarly, antihistamines are inadequately administered by way of OTC topical preparations. A lotion or cream which contains calamine, zinc oxide, menthol, and glycerin should work well.

There are no oral antihistamines marketed specifically for insect bites and stings, but several OTC capsules and tablets are available for other common ailments. These can certainly be put to good use against the swelling and itching caused by insect attacks.

Used *immediately* following an attack, these products will *prevent* much discomfort in those individuals who usually react excessively; that is, those individuals who develop large bite or sting sores that lead to local swelling and irritation. Generally, antihistamines will have little effect, except for a possible reduction in itching, after a sore has developed. Of the products available, I prefer those that contain pheniramine.

Although lice bite and cause local irritation of infected skin, this is only one aspect of their infestation. The second, and possibly more annoying and troublesome component, is the infestation itself. These pests don't leave following their biting but actually reside on the hairy parts of the body. Consequently, treating the sore does not get rid of the problem. Additional treatment is necessary.

Since the lice are difficult to see, it is wise to check for their eggs if small, itchy, red, raised sores are noted on the scalp, in the armpits, or around the groin and pubis. The eggs, "nits," are small black lumps that are attached to hair shafts. The lice, themselves, when viewed under a magnifying glass, look like small insects or crabs; thus the name "crab lice" or simply "crabs." Without the aid of a magnifying device, the small lice appear to be a tiny dark speckle, smaller than a grain of sand, resting on the skin or hair.

Fortunately, there are over-the-counter products that effectively eliminate lice and should be used when these parasites are detected. The products contain pyrethrins and piperonyl butoxide.

COMMENTS AND CAUTIONS

There are specific indications for physician-directed treatment of insect bites and stings. Spider bites that are followed by muscle cramps and weakness must be treated immediately. Don't wait to see what happens, go to your doctor.

Whenever breathing difficulty or wheezing develops after a bite or sting, an allergic reaction has probably begun. Without experienced medical assistance, the victim is in great jeopardy. Emergency room facilities and a doctor's help are definitely needed.

Fever with chills, general weakness, and hives or skin rashes should also be brought to the attention of a doctor when they follow an insect bite or sting.

INSECT STING AND BITE MEDICATIONS

Boldface: Recommended

Benadex, ointment
benzocaine 2%
phenol 1%
aluminum acetate 2%
petrolatum

Bevill's Lotion
methyl salicylate 1%
salicylic acid
ether 8%
alcohol 68%

Blueboro Bath
aluminum sulfate
calcium acetate
boric acid
blue #1

Chiggerex, ointment
benzocaine 2%
camphor 0.008%
menthol 0.005%
olive oil 0.008%
peppermint oil 0.005%
methylparaben 0.002%
clove oil 0.002%

Chiggertox Liquid
benzocaine 2.1%
benzyl benzoate 21.4%
soft soap 21.4%
alcohol 53%

Derma Medicone, ointment
benzocaine 20 mg/g
zinc oxide 137 mg/g
menthol 4.8 mg/g
8-hydroxyquinoline sulfate 10.5 mg/g
ichthammol 10 mg/g
petrolatum
lanolin
perfume

Dermoplast, spray	benzocaine 4.5% menthol 0.5% methylparaben 2% benzethonium chloride 0.1% alcohol 1.9%
Domeboro, bath	aluminum sulfate calcium acetate
Dome-Paste, bandage	zinc oxide gelatin calamine
Mediconet, pads	hamamelis water 50% glycerin 10% lanolin 0.5% methylparaben 0.15% benzalkonium chloride 0.02% perfume
Nupercainal Cream	dibucaine 0.5% acetone sodium bisulfite 0.37% washable base
Nupercainal Ointment	dibucaine 1% acetone sodium bisulfite 0.5%
Nupercainal Spray	dibucaine 0.25% alcohol 46%
Pyribenzamine, cream	tripelennamine 2% washable base
Pyribenzamine, ointment	tripelennamine 2% petrolatum
Quotane, ointment	dimethisoquin hydrochloride
Rexall First Aid Spray	benzocaine camphor methylbenzethonium chloride tyloxapol chlorothymol alcohol 4%
Soyaloid, colloid bath	soy protein polyvinyl pyrrolidene

Surfadil, cream	methapyrilene hydrochloride 2% cyclomethycaine 0.5% titanium dioxide 5%
Topic, gel	camphor menthol isopropyl alcohol 30% benzyl alcohol 5% greaseless base
Tronothane, cream, jelly	pramoxine hydrochloride 1%
Tucks, cream, pads, ointment	hamamelis water 50% glycerin 10% methylparaben 0.1% benzalkonium chloride 0.003%
Zinco Calamine	calamine 154.05 mg/30 ml zinc oxide 154.05 mg/30 ml glycerin 1.8% phenol 1%

ANTIHISTAMINES

Coricidin Tablets	aspirin 325 mg caffeine 30 mg chlorpheniramine maleate 2 mg
Coricidin Medilets	aspirin 80 mg chlorpheniramine maleate 0.5 mg
Decapryn, syrup	doxylamine succinate 6.25 mg/5 ml
Euphenex, tablet	acetaminophen 300 mg phenyltoloxamine citrate 25 mg caffeine 15 mg
Inhiston, tablet	pheniramine maleate 10 mg

ANTILICE MEDICATIONS

A 200, liquid	pyrethrins 0.165% piperonyl butoxide 2.0% deodorized kerosene 5.0% inert ingredients 92.835%

A 200, gel

pyrethrins 0.33%
piperonyl butoxide 4.00%
deodorized kerosene 5.33%
inert ingredients 90.334%

Bark, liquid

isobornyl thiocyanoacetate 4.1%
related compounds 0.9%
inert ingredients 95.0%

Cuprex, liquid

tetrahydronaphthalene 30.97%
copper oleate 0.03%
inert ingredients 69%

Rid, liquid

pyrethrins 0.30%
piperonyl butoxide 3.00%
petroleum distillates 1.20%
benzyl alcohol 2.40%
inert ingredients 93.10%

Triple X, liquid

pyrethrins 0.300%
piperonyl butoxide 3.00%
petroleum distillages 1.20%
inert ingredients 95.5%

Vonce, shampoo

pyrethrins 0.165%
piperonyl butoxide 1.65%
deordorized kerosene 1.485%
inert ingredients 96.7%

25. Insomnia

What is sleep?
Sleep is a specific state of mind and body that is characterized by interruption of sensory awareness and physical activity. It is a time of muscular relaxation, deep slow breathing, decreased heart rate, and lowered blood pressure.

Are there truly different levels of sleep?
Yes, there are. For simplicity, they can be divided into three stages.

Stage I, which can be considered light sleep, is a level somewhere between waking and sleeping. This stage occurs when someone is in the process of falling asleep or waking up.

Stage II, which is also known as medium deep sleep, predominates our sleeping pattern, comprising as much as 70 percent of all our sleeping time.

Stage III, often referred to as deep sleep, occurs about one hour after falling asleep and is associated with slow steady brain waves and great relaxation.

What is REM sleep?
REM sleep represents a specific period of Stage III sleeping time which is characterized by rapid eye movement and a short increase in the heart and breathing rate. It lasts only a few minutes to a half-hour, and may recur several times in the course of one night. Involving memory with sleep, the REM state is a time when most dreams occur.

How much sleep do we really need?
There are no specific sleep requirements since all people are different and sleeping patterns vary with age and activity.

Six hours of sleep might be perfect for one person, yet another person couldn't "survive" without ten hours. Generally, infants and young children sleep thirteen to sixteen hours each day, while teenagers sleep nine to eleven hours, and adults spend six to eight hours asleep each night. REM sleep also decreases with age and ranges from 50 percent of total sleeping time for infants to 15 percent for older adults.

What happens when we don't get enough sleep?
Aside from being in a "bad mood," nothing significant happens to our minds or bodies if we fail to get enough sleep on any one night. Performance the next day should be normal as long as motivation is maintained. The only people who might possibly suffer from short-term sleep loss are epileptics, since their chances of having a seizure increase following a sleepless night. Other people with intense or demanding jobs may also be moderately affected.

What happens to our bodies if days of sleeplessness befall us?
Since our bodies rely on sleep for revitalization, prolonged sleep loss is associated with impaired physical performance, fatigue, irritability, drowsiness, inattentiveness, and minor emotional and behavioral changes. Occasionally, extreme behavioral disorders will follow prolonged periods of sleeplessness, but there seem to be underlying psychological factors involved in such cases, and sleep loss only precipitates rather than causes the disorder.

What is insomnia?
Insomnia is a very common ailment that affects almost everyone to some degree, especially nowadays with the hectic, pressured life-styles we all are forced to lead. This problem of sleeplessness may take on different forms, but it all results in insufficient amounts of sleep to feel good. Some insomniacs may have trouble falling asleep or may be unable to stay asleep, having frequent wakings throughout the night. Others, although they actually sleep all night, believe they are really staying awake. Although everyone experi-

ences occasional sleepless nights, a true insomniac is a person who continuously fails to get the sleep he needs to function effectively the next day.

What causes insomnia?

Prolonged insomnia can be a symptom of serious underlying mental or physical illness, but transient insomnia, the occasional inability to sleep soundly, may have a variety of far less significant causes which include:

Age: As we get older our sleeping patterns change and the amount of sleep we get diminishes. Although many elderly people worry about getting less sleep than they did when they were younger, this is a natural phenomenon.

Stress and anxiety: The worries and concerns that plague us during the day can haunt us at night when we are trying to sleep. Stress and anxiety are common causes of sleeplessness.

Pain: One of the major causes of temporary insomnia is pain from any source. During the day when mental activity is directed at specific endeavors, physical discomfort may easily be ignored. However, in the evenings, at bedtime, when the mind is not occupied by the thoughts of the day, pain can attract mental attention and prevent sleep.

Change in life-style: If our daily routines are interrupted by travel or different working hours or late-night activities, our normal pattern of waking and sleeping will probably be affected. Although conditioning, getting used to the change, will quickly restore normal body functions, initially sleeplessness may occur.

Drugs: Using different drugs, such as stimulants, decongestants, and diet aids, plus food, such as coffee, cola, and tea, may promote difficulty in sleeping at night.

Physical ailments: Certain physical problems become worse at night or occur during sleep. As an example, asthma attacks are common at night and will certainly prevent restful sleep.

Distracting surroundings: Usually we sleep in a specific place and become accustomed to the surroundings of our bedrooms. Some people can sleep through the noise of city traffic; others never have to contend with such distractions. However, the addition or subtraction of a specific element to our surroundings could very easily upset our sleeping patterns and lead to temporary insomnia.

What can be done to alleviate insomnia?
Initially, an attempt must be made to discover the cause of the insomnia. If it is a constant, ongoing occurrence, underlying emotional and psychological problems, such as depression, might be the cause, in which case medical assistance is needed. Otherwise, for transient, infrequent sleepless nights, minor problems are probably the cause.

Assuming that the problem can neither be identified nor easily corrected once discovered (age, stress, change in work habits), several practices might help to relieve the accompanying insomnia.

1. Don't try to force yourself to sleep. This will never work and can only aggravate the condition. Instead, read, listen to quiet music, or possibly watch television. When a feeling of drowsiness comes on, attempt to fall asleep again.

2. Try to exercise more during the day or early evening. Physical fatigue should help you to sleep.

3. Change the room in which you sleep. Try the sofa in the living room, if no other bedrooms are available. Occasionally this type of change has a beneficial effect.

4. Avoid napping during the day or in the evening, even if you feel tired at these times. By staying awake throughout the day, your chances of having a sound sleep at night increase greatly, and your body will develop a natural rhythm of sleep and wakefulness.

Are there medications available without a prescription that will promote sleep?
Yes, several products that might aid the occasional non-sleeper are available over the counter. The drugs most often found in OTC sleep aids include scopalamine and aminoxide, a similarly related compound, plus antihistamines and mild pain relievers.

Before I discuss them, I would like to point out that these

products should not be used continuously and are not intended for the chronic insomniac. Their use is questioned by the medical and pharmacological professions, and they should only be taken when other measures to promote sleep have failed. I also want to stress the importance of removing or treating the insomnia itself. For example, if pain or physical discomfort is causing sleeplessness, take a pain-relieving drug. If heartburn or indigestion is keeping you from a good night's sleep, by all means take an antacid, or even better, eat earlier in the evening if possible. Find the cause for the insomnia and eliminate it before you take medications that aid sleep. Also, I do not recommend sleep aids for children, unless they are specifically prescribed by a physician.

How does scopalamine promote sleep?
Scopalamine reduces the electrical activity in the brain, especially in the higher centers of mental function, the cerebral cortex. It also reduces the waking effect that light has on the brain.

What are the effects of scopalamine?
Scopalamine has numerous effects on the body; effects that are sometimes unpredictable. It may cause sedation, drowsiness, and fatigue, but occasionally it will have the reverse effect of euphoria, excitement, and uneasiness, reactions that are certainly not wanted by people who are trying to sleep. Although these effects are usually related to the amount of drug that is taken (larger doses tending to cause excitement instead of sedation), not all people respond alike and some will be stimulated by small amounts of the drug. The side effects of scopalamine include dry mouth, visual disturbances, and difficulty in urinating.

How does methapyrilene promote sleep?
The mode of action of methapyrilene on the brain is not precisely known, but this compound, like other anti-histamines, produces mild drowsiness and sedation. Actually, these actions are side effects of a drug that is primarily

used to combat allergies; however, because methapyrilene is safe and can produce sleepiness, the federal Food and Drug Administration allows its use as a sleep aid.

What are other effects of methapyrilene?
Methapyrilene has the same effect as other antihistamines, including dryness of the mouth and throat, dizziness, upset stomach, and thickening of the mucus in the respiratory tract.

Because of the relative safety of antihistaminic drugs, are they safe for everyone?
No! There is no drug that is safe for everyone, not even antihistamines. Since they may have an ill effect on developing unborn babies, they should not be taken by pregnant women, nor should they be used by nursing mothers or infants. People who suffer from glaucoma, peptic ulcer, prostate enlargement, asthma, heart disease, thyroid disease, high blood pressure, or diabetes should use these drugs only as recommended by their doctor.

What about pyrilamine?
Pyrilamine is another antihistamine that is found in sleep-aid products. Its actions and effects are similar to methapryrilene; so are its hazards.

RECOMMENDED TREATMENT
Personally, I discourage the use of scopalamine or aminoxide as a sleeping aid; if a product must be used, I recommend one that is composed solely of methapyrilene or pyrilamine.

COMMENTS AND CAUTIONS
Occasional insomnia is nothing to worry about; the worst it will do is create mild irritability the following day. Continuous insomnia is another story. As mentioned previously, it can lead to serious emotional disturbances or may actually be caused by psychological problems, such

as depression, that require psychiatric attention. Please be reasonable. If you suffer from prolonged sleeplessness, avoid the use of any sleep aid and see your doctor.

A word of caution about scopalamine and aminoxide! These drugs should not be given to children unless prescribed or administered by a doctor. Since infants and youngsters are very susceptible to the effects produced by both scopalamine and aminoxide, fatal poisonings can easily occur with overdose.

These drugs should not be used by people who have glaucoma, heart disease, or enlargement of the prostate gland. Nor should they be taken with other drugs unless supervised by a physician. Again, children should not use scopalamine or aminoxide as a sleep aid!

SLEEP PROMOTIONAL DRUGS

Boldface: Recommended

Compoz, tablet	methapyrilene hydrochloride 15 mg pyrilamine maleate 10 mg
Dormin, capsule	methapyrilene hydrochoride 25 mg
Nervine, tablet (capsule-shaped)	methapyrilene hydrochloride 25 mg
Nervine, tablet (effervescent)	methapyrilene fumarate, equivalent to methapyrilene hydrochloride 25 mg
Nervine, liquid	methapyrilene fumarate, equivalent to methapyrilene hydrochloride 25 mg/5 ml
Nite Rest, capsule	methapyrilene hydrochloride 50 mg aminoxide hydrobromide 0.25 mg
Nytol, capsule	methapyrilene hydrochloride 50 mg salicylamide 380 mg
Nytol, tablet	methapyrilene hydrochloride 25 mg salicylamide 200 mg

Quiet World, tablet	methapyrilene hydrochloride 25 mg aspirin 227.5 mg acetaminophen 162.5mg
Relax-U-Caps	methapyrilene hydrochloride 25 mg
Sedacaps	methapyrilene hydrochloride 25 mg
Seedate, capsule	methapyrilene hydrochloride 25 mg aminoxide hydrobromide 0.125 mg
Sleep-Eeze, tablet	methapyrilene hydrochloride 25 mg hydrobromide 0.125 mg.
Sleepinal, capsule	methapyrilene hydrochloride 50 mg
Sominex, capsule	methapyrilene hydrochloride 50 mg aminoxide hydrobromide 0.5 mg salicylamide 200 mg
Sominex, tablet	methapyrilene hydrochloride 25 mg aminoxide hydrobromide 0.25 mg salicylamide 200 mg
Somnicaps	methapyrilene hydrochloride 25 mg
Tranquil, capsule	methapyrilene fumarate 25 mg sodium salicylate 25 mg acetaminophen 25 mg
Tranquim, capsule	methapyrilene hydrochloride 50 mg

26. Menstrual Discomfort

What is menstruation and why does it occur?
Prior to the release of an egg from the ovaries, the lining of the uterus becomes soft and fluffy, awaiting a possible conception and implantation of the fertilized egg. If pregnancy does not occur, the uterine lining (endometrium) sloughs off, bleeding begins, and a new period is started. If pregnancy does occur, bleeding does not take place because the thick, rich endometrium is sustained by pregnancy hormones and provides a well-suited environment for the growing embryo.

The changes that lead to periodic monthly bleeding, menstrual periods, are controlled by the female hormones and occur month after month in the absence of pregnancy. Periods generally begin at puberty and last until the menopause, a time of reduced hormone function.

At what specific age does menstruation normally begin?
Normally, girls about thirteen years of age begin to menstruate, but bleeding may appear in girls as young as nine or as old as sixteen. The most significant facts influencing the onset of menstruation are: the age at which menses began in the mother; health and nutrition; weight, race, and emotional stability.

How often should periods occur?
One period every twenty-eight days is the established norm, but few women are perfectly "normal." Slight variation in the length of the menstrual cycles is usually noted, even in the most regular women. Consequently, twenty-one to

thirty-five day intervals are considered acceptable. Cycles shorter or longer than these may indicate abnormal menstrual function.

How long should a period last?
Most women experience three to five days of bleeding, with the greatest amount of blood flowing early in the period. Some women, however, menstruate for as many as eight days, while others bleed for only two days.

How much blood is lost during a period?
Differences in the amount of blood lost during a period are as widespread as the other components of the menstrual cycle. Occasionally, no blood is noted, especially in women who take birth control pills, but a blood loss up to 150 milliliters (approximately one-half cup) is within normal limits.

What body changes are associated with normal menstruation?
Normally, prior to blood flow, a slight weight gain is noted in many women. This is due to an increase in the water content of the body, caused by changing female hormones. Because of this fluid retention, minor swelling of the face, hands, and feet occasionally results along with breast enlargement and tenderness. Mental changes may also occur and usually take the form of irritability and mild depression.

Although most women experience only minor difficulty during their period, some women suffer through more annoying problems. Pelvic pain and fullness can precede or extend throughout the entire period. Cramps are common and usually mild, but sporadically cause disruption of daily activities. Anxiety and tension may be marked. In more extreme cases, headaches, diarrhea, dizziness, nausea, and vomiting are noted.

What should be done for occasional menstrual discomfort?
Because menstrual discomfort is usually minor and insignificant, it should be tolerated as much as possible. Daily

activities should proceed as normal, thereby avoiding undue preoccupation with menstrual changes. Physical exercise should be increased because it promotes relaxation and reduces anxiety. A healthy diet should be maintained. By tolerating the normal mild discomfort of menstrual periods, specific treatment can be reserved for more annoying problems that might arise.

What can be done for *excessive* swelling?

The increase in female hormones that occurs with menstruation causes salt accumulation in the body. Because salt retention leads to fluid retention, water swelling of the face, hands, and feet is noted during the period. By reducing the amount of salt in her diet, a woman can avoid much of the bloating, swelling, and puffiness that is associated with her period.

Are there medications that reduce water swelling?

Yes, there are a host of prescription and nonprescription medications that reduce the water swelling associated with menstrual periods. Those found in over-the-counter menstrual products are ammonium chloride, caffeine, and pamabrom.

Ammonium chloride: Ammonium chloride works on the kidneys to increase the amount of salt and water that is eliminated from the body with urination. In appropriate dosages, it will have an acceptable short-term (two- to three-day) effect. But no OTC product contains the recommended amount, 6000 to 10000 mg. See Chapter 7, "Colds and Flus" (page 58).

Caffeine: As anyone who drinks coffee or tea will testify, caffeine causes frequent urination and thus promotes water and salt loss. Caffeine also produces mental alertness, wakefulness, and occasional restlessness. It is found in half of the OTC menstrual products. See Chapter 15, "Drowsiness and Fatigue" (pages 173-74).

Pamabrom: Pamabrom is a substance that is similar to caffeine in many respects, including its potential to relieve fluid swelling by increasing urination. Its effectiveness is approximately equal to that of caffeine.

What can be done for excessive pain and cramping?
Much of the pain and essentially all of the cramping associated with menstrual periods is due to muscular contractions of the uterus. By sitting in a bathtub filled with hot water, uterine muscles will relax and a considerable amount of discomfort will be relieved.

Are there any medications available over the counter that will also relieve cramps and pain caused by uterine contractions.?
Yes, there are basically three types of medications available.

Aspirin: Aspirin and the aspirin-like compounds, acetaminophen and phenacetin, will relieve much of the pain caused by uterine contractions. In addition, the headaches and the breast tenderness that occur with the period are alleviated with the use of these compounds. See Chapter 1, "Aches and Pains" (page 4).

Cinnamedrine: This antispasmodic agent supposedly reduces uterine cramping and, in this way, prevents pelvic pain and pressure. Although some evidence to support its effectiveness is available, general medical acceptance of this substance is lacking.

Atropine, homatropine: Both atropine and homatropine are antispasmodic drugs that reduce muscular tone and decrease cramping. However, the concentration of these substances in OTC menstrual products is insufficient to produce the desired effect.

What can be done to relieve menstrual irritability?
Menstrual irritability is difficult to control because its precise cause is unknown. It may be related to changes in the various salt concentrations of the body fluids. Psychological conditioning probably plays a contributing role as well. Regardless, without an established explanation, treatment is generally useless. Physical exercise may be beneficial and relaxing pastimes might also help to ease tension.

Can OTC medications provide some relief?
The OTC medications for menstrual irritability include two antihistamine compounds, pyrilamine and phenindamine. Both of these drugs act as mild sedatives, but the amounts present in OTC menstrual products are inadequate. Furthermore, their effectiveness in controlling the tension and irritability associated with menstrual periods is not well established.

RECOMMENDED TREATMENT
Having reviewed the current literature and numerous pharmacology texts, I recommend aspirin or acetaminophen for minor pains, and caffeine or pamabrom for the reduction of swelling. Cinnamedrine can be taken for cramps. Product selection should be based on previous experience, and those medications known to cause personal ill effects should be avoided. For nausea and vomiting, see Chapter 27 (pages 272-77).

COMMENTS AND CAUTIONS
When bleeding is prolonged and excessive, aspirin products should not be taken because they can promote increased blood loss. Instead, a doctor should be consulted. Medical consultation is also advised if pain is extreme and debilitating.

MENSTRUAL PRODUCTS

Boldface: Recommended

Aqua-Ban, tablet | ammonium chloride 325 mg
caffeine 100 mg

Cardui, tablet | salicylamide 250 mg
phenacetin 125 mg
pamabrom 25
pyrilamine maleate 12.5 mg

Cope, tablet	aspirin 421 mg caffeine 32 mg methapyrilene fumarate 12.5 mg magnesium hydroxide 50 mg aluminum hydroxide 25 mg
Femcaps, capsule	aspirin phenacetin caffeine ephedrine sulfate 8 mg atropine sulfate 0.03 mg
Femicin, tablet	salicylamide 225 mg acetaminophen 160 mg caffeine 65 mg pyrilamine maleate 15 mg homatropine methylbromide 0.5 mg
Flowaway Water 100's, tablet	potassium nitrate 171 mg uva ursi extract 98 mg buchu leaves extract 24 mg caffeine 20 mg
Fluidex, tablet	buchu leaves extract 65 mg couch grass extract 65 mg corn silk extract 32.5 mg hydrangea extract 32.5 mg
Fluidex-Plus with Diadax, tablet	buchu leaves extract 65 mg couch grass extract 65 mg corn silk extract 32.5 mg hydrangea extract 32.5 mg phenylpropanolamine hydrochloride 25 mg
Humphrey's No.11, tablet	cimicifuga pulsatilla sepia
Lydia Pinkham, tablet	Jamaica dogwood extract pleurisy root extract licorice extract ferrrus sulfate

Lydia Pinkham Vegetable Compound, Liquid	Jamaica dogwood extract pleurisy root extract licorice extract alcohol
Midol, caplet	aspirin 453.6 mg caffeine 32.4 mg cinnamedrine 14.9 mg
Odrinil, tablet	buchu leaves extract 34.4 mg uva ursi extract 34.4 mg corn silk extract 34.4 mg juniper extract 16.2 mg caffeine 16.2 mg
Pamprin, tablet	salicylamidc 250 mg phenacetin 125 mg pamabrom 25 mg pyrilamine maleate 12.5 mg
Pre-Mens Forte, tablet	ammonium chloride 500 mg caffeine 100 mg
Sunril, capsule	acetaminophen 300 mg pamabrom 50 mg pyrilamine maleate 25 mg
Trendar, tablet	acetaminophen 240 mg pamabrom 50 mg phenindamine tartrate 12.5 mg
Zodiex, tablet	phenacetin 125 mg salicylamine pamabrom 25 mg pyrilamine maleate

27. Nausea and Vomiting

What is nausea?
Nausea is a queasy sensation that heralds the approach of vomiting. It not only serves as a warning that vomiting may commence, it also protects the body. By suppressing the appetite, nausea prevents eating which would only place unneeded and potentially dangerous food in an already distressed stomach.

Where does the sensation of nausea originate?
The sensation of nausea actually originates in the base of the brain within a very specialized area called the nausea center. When stimulated by incoming nerve impulses, the nausea center alerts the rest of the brain that impending illness is at hand, and, in this way, the conscious feeling of sickness is realized.

What causes stimulation of the nausea center?
Many things cause stimulation of the nausea center. Heightened emotions, sickening smells, tastes, or sights, illness of body organs, intense pain, or unnatural body movements are just a few common causes. Each of these unpleasant conditions directs nerve impulses to different parts of the brain, and, when the impulses are strong and numerous enough to hit the nausea center, a feeling of illness results.

Does the stimulus to vomit originate in the brain also?
Yes, it does. As a matter of fact, there is a vomiting center located next to the nausea center at the base of the brain.

272

Basically the same conditions that activate the nausea center will stimulate the vomiting center, and, if the vomiting threshold is exceeded, the stomach regurgitates its contents.

A third area in the brain, the chemical receptor trigger zone, is sensitive to drugs, toxins, and poisons in the body. When these substances are present in the blood, the trigger zone will detect them, then send messages to the nausea and vomiting centers. Again, if the vomiting threshold is exceeded, the stomach contents are regurgitated. Thus, both nausea and vomiting are controlled by the nervous system.

How does the stomach empty during vomiting?
Just before vomiting commences, saliva fills the mouth, then, following a deep breath, the muscles of the belly violently contract, creating pressure within the abdomen. Vomiting occurs when the esophagus, a muscular tube which leads from the mouth to the stomach, relaxes and the stomach, which normally contracts from top to bottom during normal activities, tightens in a reverse manner, sending its contents through the esophagus and out of the mouth.

Is vomiting beneficial?
At times vomiting is beneficial, especially when poisons or toxins that could create serious illness are present within the stomach. By regurgitating these poisons, the body is protected from their harmful effects.

Other periods of vomiting, those associated with severe pain or bad headaches, for example, appear to have no protective or helpful purpose. Instead, they simply add to the anguish and anxiety already experienced by the ill person, and, in some ways, contribute to the illness.

What illnesses are associated with vomiting?
The following illnesses are associated with vomiting.

Gastritis: Gastritis, an inflammation of the stomach, is associated with nausea, vomiting, and several other symptoms including heartburn, bloating, abdominal pain, and pressure.

Gastroenteritis: Quite common in children as a cause of vomiting, gastroenteritis may lead to vomiting in adults also. This illness is an inflammation and irritation of the stomach and small bowel, frequently of viral origin. It lasts only a few days but, during that time, may produce weakness, cramps, fever, muscular aches and pains, diarrhea, loss of appetite, and headaches, along with the nausea and vomiting. Other causes of gastroenteritis, in addition to viral infections, include overindulgence in food or drink, food poisoning, bacterial and parasitic infections, food allergies, and certain medications.

Peptic ulcers: Peptic ulcers may occur in the stomach or in the first part of the small intestine, the duodenum. Pain in the upper abdomen is the most common complaint of peptic ulcer sufferers, but other ulcer symptoms—heartburn, stomach distention, weight loss, nausea, and vomiting—also occur with considerable frequency.

Intestinal obstruction: The causes of intestinal obstruction are numerous, but the symptoms are the same. Abdominal distention, cramps, visible movements of the stomach and intestines, constipation or diarrhea, pain, gas, nausea, and vomiting may take place individually or in any combination. The specific symptoms that are experienced depend on the location of the obstruction. Nausea and vomiting are most common when the obstruction occurs in the upper part of the small intestine.

Inflammation of abdominal organs: Nausea and vomiting are both associated with inflammation of the liver, gallbladder, pancreas, and kidneys. Furthermore, when pelvic organs, such as the uterus, tubes, ovaries, and urinary bladder, are irritated or infected, vomiting may also occur.

Brain disorders: Diseases which increase the pressure inside the head can produce violent vomiting. Examples of such diseases include brain tumors and strokes.

Other illnesses that affect the brain may also cause vomiting. Migraine headaches, which usually occur on one side of the head and are frequently preceded by visual or other sensory disturbances, may lead to extensive vomiting. High fevers, especially in children, produce vomiting. And, toxic substances, including drugs, can stimulate the chemical receptor trigger zone in the brain which might, in turn, act on the vomiting center and ultimately provoke regurgitation.

Emotional distress: In susceptible people, the sight of blood or possibly the excitement generated by an unexpected event may cause an exaggerated response such as vomiting. Occasionally, emotionally disturbed individuals will vomit deliberately to draw attention to themselves or to evoke sympathy from others.

Pregnancy: One of the most common causes of vomiting is pregnancy. The exact reason for the vomiting is not precisely known but may be related to pregnancy hormones that increase after conception.

Motion sickness: Within each ear there is a small, but very sensitve, organ that controls balance and equilibrium. These organs can detect subtle changes in the position or movement of the head and can relay that information to the brain. When over stimulated, they can also produce nausea and vomiting. Dizziness and light-headedness are frequent companions of the nausea and vomiting of motion sickness.

What does vomiting blood indicate?
Vomiting blood usually indicates serious disease. Peptic ulcers, tumors, severe cases of gastritis, and large bleeding veins of the stomach and esophagus that are associated with cirrhosis of the liver, can all produce debility and death through blood loss. Vomiting is common to all these ailments, and regurgitated blood should alert the ill person of the possibility of serious disease.

Can the appearance of the vomited blood indicate the site of bleeding?
Yes. Thin, bright red, regurgitated blood is probably from the esophagus or stomach. However, if this blood sits in the stomach before being vomited, it will become digested by gastric juices and then takes on a dark brown color, sometimes having the appearance of coffee grounds. If the blood is mixed with saliva, the bleeding may be from the mouth or upper respiratory tract.

What products are available to control vomiting?
There are several products available without a prescription for the control of vomiting. They fall into three categories: antihistamines, carbohydrates, and bismuth compounds.

Antihistamines: These products tend to depress the brain and reduce nerve impulses. By exerting such an effect on the nausea and vomiting centers, antihistamines help to relieve vomiting. Although there are other drugs that are more effective against vomiting, the antihistamines are the most powerful products available without a prescription, and many doctors recommend their use before going to a stronger prescription drug. Meclizine and dimenhydrinate are found in several OTC products.

Carbohydrates: Supposedly, these substances reduce vomiting by slowing down the contractions and pulsations of the stomach, although their effectiveness is not well documented. Since they are composed primarily of sugars—fructose, sucrose, and glucose—they may cause problems for diabetics and should be avoided by those people.

Bismuth compounds: The bismuth compounds are used for nausea and vomiting that is associated with overeating or other dietary indiscretions. These substances are said to work on the stomach wall, but there is inconclusive evidence that bismuth compounds exert any effect on the stomach at all. No effects on the nausea or vomiting centers in the brain are known either. Bismuth subnitrate may cause blood problems in young children, so excessive use in youngsters should be avoided.

RECOMMENDED TREATMENT

I personally think that, of all the OTC nausea and vomiting products available, the antihistamines are the best. Studies show little difference in the effectiveness of meclizine, cyclizine, or dimenhydrinate, so any one of these can be used. They are particularly effective against the nausea and vomiting of motion sickness.

People who suffer from eye pain because of glaucoma or

from urinary retention due to prostate enlargement should avoid antihistamines if possible. Pregnant women should also avoid them.

COMMENTS AND CAUTIONS

Vomiting during pregnancy should be treated by a physician because of the possible side effects that drugs exert on the developing baby. Although the warning against antihistamine use in early pregnancy has been lifted, continued drug use by pregnant women is against good judgment.

Young children and infants who develop frequent or prolonged vomiting should surely be examined by a doctor. Since babies are very susceptible to the water and nutrient losses that occur with vomiting, serious complications can quickly develop if treatment is delayed or faulty. If occasional vomiting is associated with rapid or excessive feedings in newborns, feeding procedures should be corrected and drug therapy should be avoided.

Vomiting in older children or adults that lasts more than two days, or is associated with other serious signs of illness, such as persistent headaches, abdominal pain, severe cramps, or blood, should be brought to the attention of a doctor.

VOMIT CONTROL MEDICATIONS

Boldface: Recommended

Bonine, tablet	meclizine hydrochloride 25 mg
Dramamine, tablet	dimenhydrinate 50 mg
Dramamine, liquid	dimenhydrinate 15 mg/5 ml sucrose 54% ethanol 5% flavor 0.2%
Eldodram, tablet	dimenhydrinate 50 mg
Emetrol, liquid	sugar 3.74 g/5 ml phosphoric acid 25 mg/5 ml

Marezine, tablet	cyclizine hydrochloride 50 mg
Pepto-Bismol, tablet	bismuth subsalicylate calcium carbonate aminoacetic acid
Pepto-Bismol, liquid	bismuth subsalicylate calcium carbonate
Ram, tablet	dimenhydrinate 50 mg
Trav-arex, tablet	dimenhydrinate 50 mg
Vertrol, tablet	meclizine hydrochloride 12.5 mg

28. Obesity

What is obesity?
Obesity is the excessive accumulation of fat in the body.

Why does obesity occur?
There are many causes of obesity. However, it can generally
be stated that simple, uncomplicated obesity results when
food intake exceeds the body's need.

Everything we do—thinking, walking, standing, sitting—
requires energy that our bodies must generate from the foods
we eat. If our energy requirements are low (more sitting
than walking) and our food intake is high, fat is stored in the
body and will continue to be deposited as long as *food intake
exceeds the body's need.* If the amount of food we eat is
insufficient to meet our energy needs, fat is removed from
our bodies through conversion into energy and we lose
weight.

Who suffers from obesity?
Obesity is a very common problem in the United States
because of the great wealth of our wonderful country and
the availability of almost every type of food imaginable.
Some 65 million Americans are overweight, according to
various studies. In poorer countries where food is scarce,
obesity is virtually unknown and malnutrition and starva-
tion are common medical problems. Let us count our bless-
ings and our calories.

**Why does fat accumulate in the body instead of pro-
teins or carbohydrates?**
The body has a limited capacity to store proteins and carbohydrates. These two substances are either used up imme-

diately or converted into fat and stored as fatty deposits in the body. Since fat is a high-energy substance, generating 9 calories per gram or 255 calories per ounce, it is certainly more efficiently stored than carbohydrates or proteins that contain only four calories per gram or 113 calories per ounce. This is also why fatty foods contribute greatly to obesity: they contain more calories.

Where is fat deposited?
Fat is stored throughout the body, primarily directly beneath the skin. Women tend to deposit fat around the hips, legs, and arms, while men generally become bigger around the waist, chest, and shoulders. Fat also accumulates where it cannot be seen, around the heart, between the intestines, in the liver, and among skeletal and heart muscle fibers.

What are the specific causes of obesity?
In addition to overeating, the most obvious cause, there are a variety of other contributing factors. Here are some of them.

Brain disfunction: There is a specific area in the brain, the hypothalamus, that contains two food centers. One stimulates the appetite, the other depresses it. Possibly, in some individuals, these two control centers work incorrectly so that a constant hunger results, and overeating leads to obesity.

Pituitary alterations: Another specialized part of the brain, the pituitary gland, produces hormones which relate to hunger and food intake. Obesity is occasionally associated with pituitary problems and the insufficient production of pituitary hormones that also lead to a variety of additional physical and emotional complications.

Diabetes: Questionably a cause of obesity but certainly related to excessive weight, diabetes is a disease associated with abnormal utilization of sugar in the body.

Thyroid disease: The thyroid gland produces specific hormones that control the metabolic rate, or the rate food is converted into energy. If excessive amounts of thyroid hormone are produced, food is rapidly utilized and much food energy is converted to heat. With decreased thyroid hormone production, the metabolic rate is decreased, body energy needs are reduced, and food is burned up more slowly. Thus, fat may be stored rather than burned as body fuel. A decrease in thyroid hormone production, thyroid insufficiency, is also associated with poor memory, slow reflexes, coarse dry skin, and the inability to withstand cold temperatures, as well as obesity.

Old age: As we get older several things that contribute to obesity happen to us. We become less active and therefore require fewer calories to sustain our activities. There is a general decrease in our metabolic rate which in turn reduces our calorie need. We also develop a finer appreciation for food which causes us to eat more. All these factors lead to a *food intake that exceeds the body's need,* and we get fatter.

Cushing's disease: Unlike the thyroid disease and pituitary changes that result in obesity, Cushing's disease is a hormone problem resulting from an *increase* in hormones produced by the adrenal glands, small glands that rest on top of the kidneys. With this disease, fat is distributed abnormally and in excessive amounts around the belly, across the upper back, and in the cheeks of the face. Other characteristics of Cushing's disease include poor wound healing, excessive bruising, thin irregular hair growth, and purple skin discolorations which appear similar to "stretch marks."

Reduction in sex hormones: Sex hormones relate indirectly to obesity. At puberty, a time of accelerated sex hormone production, young boys and girls usually experience a loss in weight. During the menopause, when sex hormone production from the ovaries and testicles decreases, an increase in weight is frequently noted.

Hereditary factors: Like so many other medical problems, obesity has roots in our ancestry. If one of our parents is overweight, we stand a greater chance of becoming fat. If both of our parents are obese, the possibility doubles. In fact, 80 percent of children with two obese parents will experience weight problems themselves.

Psychological factors: No doubt many obese people have an increased desire to eat because of psychological problems.

Dissatisfaction with friends, associates, and possibly even with themselves, drives them to seek satisfaction through eating. Depression and anxiety frequently give rise to overeating and thus can lead to obesity, too

How can I tell if I am overweight?
For the most part, we know when we are overweight. Our clothes become a bit too tight, we feel uncomfortable, we look flabby, and of course we weigh more. One simple rule of thumb is to weigh roughly what you did when you were twenty-five, assuming you had a normal body build at that time. Another way to determine "ideal weight" is to use a common weight chart which suggests an acceptable weight for your size and build. Although these charts are not perfect, they provide a good average.

Why aren't weight charts perfect?
The charts provide an *average* "ideal weight," but none of us is average; we are all special and unique. Therefore, it is possible to be trim even though the charts say you are overweight, especially if you have a muscular physique. Vice versa, it is also possible to be overweight when the charts say you are normal if you have an excessive amount of fat in proportion to your bone and muscle structure.

Is it true that some people have more fat cells than others and this is why they are fat?
Yes, it is true; some people do have more fat cells than other people, possibly as a result of overfeeding during infancy or maybe because of hereditary factors, but this does not mean they will be overweight. Fat will only be deposited in these cells if *food intake exceeds the body's need.* Therefore, if a person with twice the normal number of fat cells eats the proper amount of food, fat will not accumulate within these cells and they will stay slim. Whereas, a person with a normal number of fat cells will cause these cells to become greatly enlarged if he or she eats excessively. Thus, it is not necessarily the number of fat cells in the body that makes a person obese, it is the amount of fat within these cells.

How does obesity affect the body?

Being overweight affects more than just your appearance; it alters your entire body, inside and out. Fat or fattylike substances accumulate in and around all of the internal organs, frequently affecting their performance. The heart and lungs must work overtime to supply the overweight body with oxygen and nutrients, while thick pads of fat actually restrict vital movements, making the work even more difficult. The liver and gallbladder must also work harder to supply the bile needed to digest fatty foods, that are usually abundant in the diet of the obese. And, to make matters worse, gallbladder disease itself is much more frequent among the overweight.

The same is true about high blood pressure, hardening of the arteries, and diabetes. Each of these conditions is worsened by obesity and, in some cases, actually caused by obesity. Frequently, by dieting and losing weight, these disorders may either be corrected or greatly improved.

Pregnant women will note that obesity leads to prolonged, difficult labor which may cause serious problems for both mother and baby. Maternal and infant deaths are certainly more common among overweight women and, even if the delivery is uncomplicated, the babies of obese women generally weigh more, have an increased proportion of fat cells in their bodies, and stand a greater chance of being overweight themselves.

Thus, obesity affects the entire body and all of its functions, not just the appearance.

What should be done?

If obesity is the result of overeating and is not caused by specific contributing disease states, it can be corrected by a change in life-style which includes a change in diet. A sensible diet, in my opinion, should be maintained constantly throughout your life, not just for the short period of time in which you attempt to lose a few pounds. Let's face facts, if dieting effects a weight loss but the diet is abandoned when the desired weight is achieved, chances are you will quickly become overweight again as your old eating habits return. Dieting should be a way of life, forever.

With this in mind, what corrections should be made? What constitutes a sensible diet?
First, it is important to eat a variety of foods that provide the proteins, vitamins, and minerals you need for normal body maintenance. Needless to say, these foods should be low in calories. Here are some suggestions.

1. Initially, the quantity of food eaten should be reduced to about 1000 calories daily while you are losing weight, then raised to the amount needed to sustain your new "trim" weight. This will vary from individual to individual, but a simple bathroom scale will tell you if you are again eating too much. Make necessary corrections immediately.

2. Restrict your consumption of red meat, and fill your protein requirements with fish or fowl. These protein sources are lower in calories than beef or pork and can be eaten more frequently. Four times per week is sufficient.

3. Use a calorie chart to tell you what foods are high in calories. Avoid the high calorie foods and incorporate more low calorie foods into your diet. This should be easy, since there are hundreds of low calorie foods you already like.

4. Concentrate primarily on salads and vegetables. These are low in calories and provide the bulk that is satisfying and the vitamins and minerals that are essential.

5. Except for one glass of fruit or vegetable juice each day, replace other fluids with water.

6. Take a vitamin and mineral supplement daily.

7. Try to eat two small meals each day. I usually have juice and coffee in the morning, along with my vitamins and minerals. At lunch, I'll eat a small salad and a small serving of vegetables. Then, at dinnertime, I'll have a couple of vegetables and a soup, or a small piece of chicken or fish and one vegetable. I constantly change vegetables, trying to consume a different type each day, thereby obtaining the nutritional benefit of each. Water is the only beverage I drink during my meals.

If you follow the above suggestions, you can lose weight

and still be satisfied. You can also be assured that you are getting the nutrients your body needs.

Many weight reduction programs have received great popularity these days and have demonstrated both success and failure in causing and maintaining weight loss. Unfortunately, some of them can be extremely dangerous to your well-being, especially "fasting" diets, total protein diets, and "fat" diets. Your personal doctor can best provide a diet suitable to your particular needs, and he or she should be consulted if you intend to try something drastic. The 1000-calorie mixed food diet mentioned above is certainly one of the safest diets that anyone can implement themselves.

What about exercise?
Exercise is not only helpful in losing weight, it also tones muscles, conditions the heart and lungs, strengthens bones and sharpens the mind. I am a great proponent of exercise. Understandably, it takes a lot of exercise to lose a little weight. Running 12 minutes or walking for 20 minutes will burn away about 200 calories. At that rate it would take 3½ hours of solid running or 6 hours of vigorous walking to burn 3600 calories and thus lose 1 pound of fat.

One suggestion is to exercise *instead* of eating between meals. Whenever the desire to snack pops into your head, jump rope in the living room or walk around the block instead of walking to the refrigerator. Because vigorous physical exertion occasionally depresses the appetite, not only will you burn up 200 calories, you might also avoid consuming another 500 calories in snacks.

Who should attempt to lose weight on their own?
Just about everyone can initiate their own weight reduction program. However, a meeting with a doctor is highly recommended for people who must lose a lot of weight, say 25 pounds or more. Large weight gains may be associated with significant medical problems, and large weight losses can severely alter the body's chemistry and function. A physician's evaluation assures good health at the beginning and end of the diet. People who have gained a few pounds

because of overeating and lack of exercise can certainly implement a personal diet without a doctor's assistance, assuming that the diet is sensible.

What are some aids to weight control?
Here is a basic summary of the most widely known methods of controlling weight.

Hormone therapy: When obesity is the result of hormone deficiencies (only your doctor could prove this for sure), hormone therapy should be considered as proper treatment.

Bulk producers: Bulk producers are substances which are used to promote a feeling of fullness after meals, but their effectiveness in causing weight reduction is questionable. Several products are available over the counter, but a low-calorie meal which includes "high bulk" foods would probably be just as effective and certainly more natural.

Appetite-depressant drugs: There are no drugs which act specifically to make people lose weight, but there are medications available which help reduce appetite. These are known as anorexic drugs and include many different agents that are related to amphetamines. How they exert their effects on appetite is debatable, but several studies have shown that they do reduce the desire to eat.

Local anesthetics: Drugs which are used to numb the mouth and possibly reduce the sense of taste have been used in weight reduction programs. Since it is thought that certain obese people have highly sensitive and well-developed taste buds, these products might be of some assistance in losing weight by making foods tasteless and, therefore, less appealing.

Artificial sweeteners: The reason for using artificial sweeteners is obvious: they allow foods to be sweetened yet add no calories to the diet.

Diet foods: There are liquid, powdered, and cookielike food products that have a mixture of protein, carbohydrate, and fat, plus vitamins and minerals. These are used in place of meals to restrict food intake and to maintain a low calorie diet. However, when used with food, as a diet supplement, they will actually promote weight gain.

Another popular diet food is digested protein, which is consumed in place of meals. However, this can be an extremely dangerous way to lose weight and, in my opinion, always requires a doctor's supervision.

RECOMMENDED TREATMENT

Bulk producers, appetite-depressant drugs, local anesthetics, artificial sweeteners, and diet food products are all available without a prescription.

Bulk producers include agar, carboxymethylcellulose, karaya gum, methylcellulose, and psyllium mucilloid. These are available in capsules, tablets, powders, and wafers. Although it is difficult to evaluate the effectiveness of specific bulk producers or the entire product line, I do believe the powder form is the safest because the possibility of intestinal obstruction caused by wafers, tablets, and capsules is virtually absent.

The only appetite-depressant drug available without a prescription is phenylpropanolamine. Supplied in combination products with caffeine, vitamins, minerals, and numerous other ingredients, phenylpropanolamine will produce a decrease in appetite by either a direct action on the appetite center in the brain or possibly through mood elevation and general stimulation. With time, the effects of this drug will diminish; and when this happens, the product should not be taken for a couple of weeks, then started again if needed. Since most of the appetite depressants are combination products that are loaded with unneeded and possibly unwanted ingredients, I recommend one that contains phenylpropanolamine and as few other substances as possible. I think that caffeine is an acceptable additional ingredient and believe that it will also help reduce the appetite.

Benzocaine is the common local anesthetic used in diet aids which take the form of gums and candies. In addition, benzocaine is also found in some oral appetite depressants produced in capsule and tablet form. Since it has no established antiappetite effect on the stomach when taken internally, I see no need to use this drug in this manner. However, when used as a candy or gum, in an attempt to numb the mouth and decrease taste, it may help the person who eats and eats and eats because everything "tastes so good." I recommend the cheapest product that contains the fewest additional ingredients.

Since the removal of cyclamates from the market, the only artificial sweetener still available in food and drug stores is saccharin. However other products are currently being developed. Saccharin contains no calories yet is approximately 400 times sweeter than sugar. I think it can be effectively used by dieters to replace sugar and reduce caloric intake, but it should be used wisely and sparingly. Excessive use of saccharin has been associated with bladder tumors in fetal mice, so the federal Food and Drug Administration is presently reevaluating its disposition. For this reason it should not be used by pregnant women.

The diet foods that you eat will depend on your particular diet and must vary accordingly. Those that are available contain numerous ingredients with different proportions of proteins, carbohydrates, and fats or oils. Personally, I would rather eat a 250- to 350-calorie meal than a can of diet food. I also think it is healthier and more natural to do so.

COMMENTS AND CAUTIONS
Better than any drug or diet food, willpower and determination are the most effective means of losing weight. By implementing a sensible diet and exercise program, you will definitely lose excessive pounds if you stick to it long enough; don't despair or become discouraged, your efforts will be rewarded in the end.

If you are able to control your weight without dietary aids, you eliminate any possible drug reaction or complication. For instance, the possibility of allergic reactions to benzocaine is nonexistent if this local anesthetic is not consumed. Since the concommitant use of phenylpropanolamine and the monoamine oxidase inhibitor drugs that are used in depression can critically escalate blood pressure, the danger of this happening is never realized when the products are not mixed. Similarly, by avoiding caffeine, the ill effects that this drug has on the cardiovascular system can never occur.

This is not to say that these products should never be taken, it merely indicates that their use should be select and discreet, their side effects should always be considered, and the duration of their consumption should be as short as possible. These principles apply to all drug therapies.

WEIGHT CONTROL MEDICATIONS
Boldface: Recommended

APPETITE SUPPRESSANTS

Anorexin, capsule

phenylpropanolamine hydrochloride 25 mg
caffeine 100 mg
carboxymethylcellulose 50 mg
ascorbic acid 20 mg
niacinamide 6 mg
thiamine 1 mg
riboflavin 1 mg
pyridoxine hydrochloride 0.33 mg
pantothenate 0.33 mg
cyanocobalamin 0.33 mcg
vitamin A 1667 IU
vitamin D 133 IU

Appedrine, tablet

phenylpropanolamine hydrochloride 25 mg
caffeine 100 mg
carboxymethylcellulose 50 mg
ascorbic acid 20 mg
niacinamide 7 mg
thiamine 1 mg
riboflavin 1 mg
pyridoxine hydrochloride 0.33 mcg
pantothenate 0.33 mg
cyanocobalamin 0.33 mcg
vitamin A 1667 IU
vitamin D 133 IU

Dexatrim, capsule	phenylpropanolamine hydrochloride 50 mg caffeine 200 mg
Diet-Trim, tablet	phenylpropanolamine hydrochloride carboxymethylcellulose benzocaine
Grapefruit Diet Plan with Diadax, tablet	phenylpropanolamine hydrochloride 10 mg ascorbic acid 10 mg vitamin E 3.6 mg natural grapefruit extract 16.6 mg
Grapefruit Diet Plan with Diadax Vitamin Fortified Continuous Action, capsule	phenylpropanolamine hydrochloride 30 mg ascorbic acid 30 mg vitamin E 11 mg natural grapefruit extract 50 mg
Hungrex, capsule	phenylpropanolamine hydrochloride 25 mg
Nature's Trim Plan with Diadax, tablet	phenylpropanolamine hydrochloride 75 mg lecithin 125 mg pyridoxine hydrochloride 21 mg cider vinegar 25 mg iodine 0.15 mg
Odrinex, tablet	phenylpropanolamine hydrochloride 25 mg caffeine 50 mg methylcellulose 50 mg
Prolamine, capsule	phenylpropanolamine hydrochloride 35 mg caffeine 140 mg
Permathene-12, capsule	phenylpropanolamine hydrochloride 75 mg caffeine 140 mg
Propadrine, capsule	phenylpropanolamine hydrochloride 25 mg

Spantrol, capsule	phenylpropanolamine hydrochloride 75 mg caffeine 150 mg carboxymethylcellulose 135 mg ascorbic acid 30 mg niacinamide 10 mg iron 10 mg benzocaine 9 mg riboflavin 1.2 mg thiamine 1 mg pyridoxine hydrochloride 1 mg
Two-Step, tablet	lactose sugar carboxymethylcellulose demineralized whey dehydrogenated vegetable oil magnesium stearate citric acid flavors
Vita-Slim, capsule	phenylpropanolamine hydrochloride 50 mg lecithin 300 mg ascorbic acid 30 mg niacinamide 10 mg pyridoxine hydrochloride 10 mg iron 9 mg pantothenate 5 mg riboflavin 0.85 mg thiamine 0.75 mg folic acid 0.2 mg kelp 75 mg cyanocobalamin 3 mcg vitamin A 2500 IU vitamin E 15 IU

BULK PRODUCING PRODUCTS

Dex-a-Diet Plan Formula, capsule	carboxymethylcellulose 200 mg vitamins minerals

Diet-Aid, tablet	carboxymethylcellulose 100 mg alginic acid 200 mg sodium bicarbonate 70 mg
Effersyllium, powder	psyllium hydrocolloid 3000 mg/7 g
Konsyl, powder	blond psyllium 100%
L.A. Formula, powder	blond psyllium 50%
Melozets, wafer	methylcellulose flour sugar
Metamucil, powder	psyllium mucilloid 50% dextrose 50%
Metamucil Instant Mix, powder packet	psyllium mucilloid 3.7 g sodium bicarbonate citric acid
Reducets, capsule	methylcellulose 100 mg benzocaine 5 mg vitamins minerals

ARTIFICIAL SWEETENERS

NectaSweet, tablet	saccharin 30 mg
Ril-Sweet, liquid	saccharin sodium 3.3%
Sucaryl Sodium, tablet	saccharin sodium 5 mg
Sucaryl Sodium, liquid	saccharin sodium 0.8%
Superose, tablet	saccharin 2.5% propylene glycol 7% benzoic acid 0.35% methyl paraben 0.035%
Sweeta, tablet	saccharin 15 mg
Sweeta, liquid	saccharin 14 mg/2 drops

Sweetaste, tablet   saccharin 15 mg/60 ml

Sweet 'N Low,   lactose
powder   saccharin 40 mg/pk

LOW-CALORIE CANDY

Ayds, soft candy
- corn syrup
- sugar
- sweetened condensed skim milk
- partially hydrogenated soybean oil
- tribasic calcium phosphate
- emulsifier
- soya flour
- invert sugar
- salt
- whey protein concentrate
- soybean lecithin
- vanilla flavor
- ferrous sulfate
- niacinamide
- vitamin A palmitate
- pyridoxine hydrochloride
- thiamine mononitrate
- riboflavin
- folic acid
- cyanocobalamin
- cocoa
- chocolate

Dex-A-Dict, capsule, tablet
- glucose
- vitamins

Slim-Line Candy, caramel
- methylcellulose 45 mg
- benzocaine 8 mg
- corn syrup
- condensed milk
- sugar
- whey
- corn syrup solids
- coconut oil
- cocoa
- chocolate
- salt
- glyceryl monostearate
- soya lecithin
- flavoring

Slim-Line Candy,
hard candy

methylcellulose 45 mg
benzocaine 8 mg
sugar
corn syrup
citric acid
flavoring

Slim-Mint, chewing
gum

methylcellulose 45 mg
sugar 1.45 g
benzocaine 8 mg
oils 3350 ppm

29. Poisoning

How common are poisonings in the United States?

Poisonings are a common problem in the United States, affecting over 1 million people each year. Of the total number of poison victims, approximately 900,000 are children, and the great majority of these children are preschoolers under five years of age.

About 3,000 deaths occur in the United States each year as a result of the 1 million poisonings. Roughly one-half of these deaths are intentional, the result of successful suicide attempts. The others are accidental and involve about twice as many children as adults.

What products commonly cause poisoning?

Drugs are the most common poisons: they are involved in about 50 percent of all cases. At the present time, minor tranquilizers such as Valium and Librium head the list, followed closely by the barbiturates. Salicylate compounds, primarily aspirin, and antidepressant drugs are also frequently abused. Furthermore, mixing the above drugs is common practice today, and when taken with alcoholic beverages, drug combinations can prove particularly lethal.

Household products, such as chlorine bleach, pine oil, furniture polish, washing soda, and the like, are occasional poisons. And, workshop chemicals which range from paint, turpentine, and lye to gasoline, kerosene, and acid take many lives each year. Insecticides are also common poisons.

How can you tell if a person has been poisoned?

Occasionally, identification of a poison victim can be made either by observing the poisoning, by speaking to the victim, or by finding empty bottles or containers around the stricken individual. However, this is not always the case; many poisonings are discovered only after extensive medical investigation.

Victims may be found unconscious with depressed breathing or a reduced heart rate. Convulsions sometimes occur. The exact reaction depends on the substance that is responsible for the poisoning, the amount of intake, and the time that has passed since the poisoning took place. In some cases, the only tip-off to a poisoning might be a recognizable odor on the breath or skin, the residue of chemicals around the mouth, or unmistakable remnants of poisons on clothing. Look for clues.

The more common symptoms of poisoning include stomach or intestinal aches and pains, nausea, vomiting, and diarrhea. These symptoms are seen most frequently with oral poisoning, but they can result from any intoxication.

Can poisonings be prevented?
Absolutely. Here are four sound preventive measures that everyone should learn.

1. By properly labeling any potentially dangerous drug or chemical, the possibility of accidental misuse is greatly reduced. Original bottles or cans will promote easy recognition of poisonous substances and should always be used in preference to catchall containers. A caution or warning should be printed on any known poison.

2. Keeping drugs and hazardous substances out of childrens' reach will prevent many poisonings, but making sure these products are out of sight is even better. Since children are inquisitive and curious, they might struggle to obtain visible poisons, but substances that are out of sight are also out of mind.

3. Drug companies and other industries are aware of the potential dangers of their products. In order to minimize these dangers, they have invented a great variety of safety containers with intricate locking tops. Although no safety device is fool- or child-proof, any precautionary measure reduces the chance of accidental childhood intoxication.

4. Education is a powerful tool that can easily be used to prevent poisonings. By teaching children the hazards of many substances, by training personnel in the proper handling of poison victims, by instructing parents in safety procedures, and by informing friends of potentially dangerous situations, many poisonings can be prevented.

What procedures will aid poison victims?

Poison victims are most properly cared for by first aid treatments and a call to the doctor, hospital, police, or rescue squad. If a poison is ingested or swallowed, the victim should be given water to drink. By diluting the poison, toxic effects will be reduced and absorption from the stomach will be slowed down. Once the water has been drunk, the victim should be made to vomit in an attempt to remove the poisons from the stomach. Vomiting should *not* be induced, however, if the sufferer is unconscious or having a seizure because of the possibility of breathing in the contents of the stomach and suffocating. Vomiting also should be avoided if the swallowed poison is a strong acid or alkali, kerosene or gasoline. These substances will cause additional damage to the esophagus, throat, and mouth if regurgitated; therefore, they are more properly neutralized with milk and removed by a doctor with a stomach tube.

If poisonous fumes or gases are inhaled, the first aid procedures change accordingly. The victim should be removed from the dangerous area and provided with fresh clean air. To aid breathing, tight clothing should be removed or loosened and artificial respiration should be initiated, if and when the sufferer stops breathing on his own.

Toxic substances on the skin or in the eyes should be removed as quickly as possible with plenty of fresh water. Soap may be used on the skin. Contact lenses should be promptly withdrawn from the eyes and contaminated clothing should be quickly removed from the body in order to avoid additional contact with the toxic substance. Again, as in all poison cases, professional assistance is of utmost importance, and a call for immediate help is essential to the proper care and treatment of the victim.

RECOMMENDED TREATMENT

The only medication that should be given to a poison victim is syrup of ipecac, a substance that will induce vomiting. Its use is restricted to poisonings where vomiting is appropriate *first aid* therapy. However, it is not intended to replace essential medical treatment. Syrup of ipecac may be purchased over the counter.

Consider this also. If vomiting is indicated and there is no syrup of ipecac immediately available, use your finger. By wiggling your fingers in the back of the victim's throat, vomiting should occur promptly. If it doesn't, you probably aren't sticking your fingers deep enough into the throat. Don't give up until you have achieved your objective. In many cases vomiting will save the victim's life.

COMMENTS AND CAUTIONS

Once again I must remind you: vomiting can be lifesaving when induced at the proper time; otherwise, it might be life threatening.

Unconscious or convulsing victims *must not* be made to vomit, and corrosive substances like acids, alkalis, or drain cleaners *should not* be regurgitated. By forcing vomiting under the above circumstances, more harm than good will surely result.

30. Psoriasis

How common is psoriasis?
Psoriasis is a disease of the skin that afflicts approximately 2 percent of the population of the United States or about 4½ million people.

What are the characteristics of this ailment?
The skin lesions of psoriasis have a very distinct appearance. Although they may vary greatly in size, from sores less than 1 inch in diameter to large patches several inches across, they all have a thick scaly character. When the sores are new, they are flat and pink but, in time, they enlarge and thicken at the center with large silvery scales. Surrounding each sore is a thin red border which lies in direct contrast to the scaly silvery centers.

While the face is seldom involved, the first signs of psoriasis usually appear on the scalp. Extension from the scalp to any irritated part of the body is the rule, but spread can be quite unpredictable and sporadic. Favorite sites of additional involvement include elbows and knees, chest and lower back, pubis and groin. Fingernail involvement is fairly common too, resulting in discoloration and deformity of the nail. When the nails are affected, the disease process begins along the skin borders but ultimately involves the entire nail. Thick scales form and gradually lift the nail off the finger, producing pits and grooves in the raised nail and imparting a pink orange color to it. The finger tips may be extremely tender.

Are there any predisposing factors to this disease?
Yes, there are. Since 25 percent of the offspring of psoriasis sufferers will have this ailment, a genetic inheritance is

likely, with men and women being equally affected. Once the disease is contracted, it generally becomes worse during the cold, damp, dismal months of winter, during periods of emotional stress, or with excessive eating. It is not contagious.

At what age does psoriasis appear?

The age distribution of psoriasis is broad: people between ten and fifty are most frequently stricken. Children characteristically develop a special form of this disease, called guttata psoriasis, which begins as numerous small, one-half to one-quarter inch, red encrusted sores that expand and blend into the larger, and more characteristic silver plaques. Occurrence frequently follows upper respiratory infections and tonsillitis in the child. Guttata psoriasis may also commence in older women after a pregnancy and delivery. Otherwise, the more common form of psoriasis is prevalent among older individuals.

How long does the disease last?

Psoriasis is a lifelong ailment that varies greatly in its severity and course. Sometimes sores may quickly disappear, leaving only a pale area on the skin as a telltale marker. At other times, lesions can persist for years as thick scaly skin patches that cause anxiety and self-consciousness in the sufferer. New sores can arise at any time.

Can psoriasis be cured?

Most physicians agree that psoriasis cannot be cured but, with adequate treatment, improvement is definitely possible. If the condition can be temporarily arrested, many people will remain disease-free for prolonged periods of time and truly seem completely well.

Can psoriasis be adequately self-treated with nonprescription drugs?

The answer to this question relates to the severity of the disease. For mild early eruptions and small chronic sores, self-treatment with OTC products will prove beneficial.

However, for larger lesions and extensive involvement of the entire body, a dermatologist's evaluation and therapy is more apropos.

Self-medication should be aggressively directed at newly formed eruptions, because these are most easily treated and arrested. The older, thicker, more unsightly lesions can possibly be averted if self-treatment is initiated in time.

What medications for psoriasis can be purchased without a prescription?

The OTC medications for psoriasis include shampoos, creams, lotions, and solutions containing allantoin, salicylic acid, sulfur, and wood or coal tar. For specific information regarding the mode of action and effectiveness of these compounds, refer to Chapter 12, "Dandruff" (pages 146-47).

How should psoriasis be treated?

Here are some basic rules to follow when self-treating psoriasis.

Early minor eruptions: When a scalp or body eruption is first noted, treatment should simply consist of washing the sore with a zinc soap or shampoo. Then, a soothing body cream or lotion should be applied to each individual sore. Normal daily activity and a good diet should be maintained; overexertion should be avoided.

Mild scaling lesions: Mild scaling lesions are best treated by removing the skin flakes with salicylic acid shampoo and a washcloth, although scrubbing to the point of irritation is not desirable. Each sore should then be covered with a mild (2–3 percent) salicylic acid, (2–5 percent) coal tar cream or lotion, that is applied by gentle rubbing.

Moderate scaling lesions: Tar baths often prove helpful when combined with salicylic acid and coal tar soaps and shampoos. Scales should be removed with gentle washing and scrubbing, then coal tar paste or cream should be applied directly to individual sores.

Since exposure to sunlight or ultraviolet light is beneficial, the daily use of a sun lamp is recommended. Radiation must cover the entire body, and initial exposure to any particular area should not exceed three to five minutes. In time, extended exposure can be tolerated in an attempt to achieve light tanning, but early prolonged use of the lamp will result in dangerous, undesirable burning. Dark goggles should always be worn during therapy.

Because anxiety and emotional stress aggravate this condition, rest and relaxation should be sought. A gentle antihistamine sedative will provide light sedation during troubled times and will also relieve the slight itching that can accompany psoriasis sores.

Large, heavily scaled patches: These lesions should be treated by a dermatologist.

RECOMMENDED TREATMENT

Salicylic acid and coal tars are effective when used early in the course of this ailment. If a new lesion is noted, direct therapy at it immediately. Don't let it enlarge and get out of hand.

Generally, the higher the concentration of active ingredients, the more effective the medication. Choose your products wisely and use them conscientiously.

COMMENTS AND CAUTIONS

Where self-medication is tried without much success (psoriasis can be stubborn), see your physician. And, if anxiety or emotional problems complicate and heighten psoriasis outbreaks, professional assistance is probably needed. It will help more than just the skin trouble.

ECZEMA OR PSORIASIS MEDICATIONS

Boldface: Recommended

Alma Tar, bath	juniper tar 35%
Alma Tar, shampoo	juniper tar 4% polyoxyethylene ethers edetate sodium sulfonated castor oil coconut oil triethanolamine

Alphosyl, lotion,
cream

coal tar 5%
allantoin 2%
hydrophilic base

Balnetar, water-
dispersible

coal tar 2.5%
mineral oil
lanolin oil

DHS Tar, shampoo

coal tar 0.5%
cleansing agents

**Diasporal-Tar,
cream**

tar distillate 5%
salicylic acid 2%
sulfur 3%
isopropyl alcohol

Epidol, liquid

coal tar 18%
salicylic acid 3%

Estar, gel

coal tar 5%
hydroalcoholic gel

Ionil T, shampoo

coal tar 5%
salicylic acid 2%
polyoxyethylene ethers
benzalkonium chloride
alcohol

Kay-San, cream

coal tar
allantoin
resorcinol
sodium salicylate
chloroxylenol

Keralyt Gel

salicylic acid 6%
propylene glycol
alcohol
cellulose

Lavator, bath oil

tar distillate 25%

L.C.D., cream

coal tar 5.8%

L.C.D., solution

coal tar 100%

Mazon, cream	coal tar 0.87% salicylic acid 1% resorcinol benzoic acid
Mazon, shampoo	coal tar 3% sulfur 1%
Oxipor, lotion	coal tar salicylic acid benzocaine alcohol
Packer's Pine Tar Soap	pine tar 6% soap
Pentrax, shampoo	coal tar 8.75% detergents
Polytar, soap, shampoo	tars 1%(juniper, pine, and coal) surface active cleansers
Polytar, bath oil	tars 25% (juniper, pine, and coal)
Poslam, ointment	tar distillate salicylic acid sulfur phenol zinc oxide menthol lanolin
Pragmatar, cream	cetyl alcohol–coal tar 4% salicylic acid 3% sulfur 3%
Psorelief, cream	coal tar allantoin isopropyl myristate psoralen
Psorex, shampoo	coal tar 2% allantoin 0.2% surface active cleansers

Psorex Medicated, cream	coal tar 0.50% allantoin 0.25% silicone surface active cleansers
Psorex Medicated, shampoo	coal tar 0.50% allantoin 0.20% lanolin protein surface active cleansers
Supertah, ointment	coal tar 0.25% zinc oxide starch
Tarbonis, cream	coal tar 5% hydrophilic base
Tar-Doak, lotion	tar distillate
Tarpaste	tar distillate 5% zinc oxide
Tarsum, shampoo	coal tar solution 10% salicylic acid 5%
Tegrin, cream, lotion, shampoo	coal tar 5% allantoin 0.2%
Tersa-Tar, shampoo	tar distillate 3%
Vanseb-T, shampoo	coal tar 5% salicylic acid 1% sulfur 2% sodium lauryl sulfate sodium stearate fatty alkylolamide condensate protein polyethylene glycol 75 lanolin silicone-glycol-copolymer imidazolidinylurea

Vanseb-T Tar, shampoo	coal tar 5% salicylic acid 1% sulfur 2% proteins surface active cleansers
Zetar, ointment, lotion	coal tar 2% zinc oxide talc
Zetar, shampoo	coal tar 1% chloroxylenol

31. Seborrhea

How can seborrhea be recognized?
People with seborrhea, and they number in the millions, complain of oily skin and greasy hair. Their skin sometimes appears thicker than normal, and enlarged pores are usually conspicuous. Most commonly, the face and scalp are involved because these areas of the body are abundant with sebaceous glands (the small skin glands that produce oily secretions).

How does one develop seborrhea?
In a great number of cases, seborrhea is inherited. Although it does appear in association with certain nervous disorders like Parkinsonism and epilepsy, this association is far less common. Regardless, it is related to the increase in sebaceous activity that develops at the time of puberty and, no doubt, is influenced by the sex hormones that flow at this time, especially testosterone, the male hormone. For this reason, men are more affected by seborrhea than women. Because the condition starts at puberty, children are spared. Those people who will ultimately develop seborrhea notice its beginnings in the early teens and its peak severity between the ages of eighteen and twenty-eight. Fortunately, seborrhea will spontaneously disappear or improve, but the time required for this to happen is quite variable. Frequently, the condition will flare during periods of stress.

What are the complications of seborrhea?
In many people, seborrhea is complicated by acne, seborrheic dermatitis, infections, facial discoloration, and noticeable enlargement of sebaceous glands.

Since increased sebaceous activity is a causal factor in the development of acne, it is reasonable to expect seborrhea sufferers to have acne skin blemishes in combination with their oily skin, and this frequently does occur. In addition, because sebaceous oil can be turned into a strong irritant by bacteria normally present on the body surface, inflammation of the skin can result. When present, seborrheic dermatitis is characterized by large, oily, yellow flakes that build up, then detach themselves from the face, eyelids, eyebrows, scalp, and body. The underlying skin is red and irritated. Bacteria frequently take advantage of the skin irritation, and, consequently, infection is common, resulting in further inflammation and pus.

The skin discoloration of seborrhea is a feature that sometimes arises in association with Parkinson's disease or other neurologic diseases. It appears on the face and develops as a brownish mask surrounding the eyes.

Occasionally, sebaceous glands will enlarge sufficiently enough to be noticed under the skin, appearing as small yellowish lumps that form across the forehead and temples or along the cheeks and nose. Men grow these sebaceous nodules more frequently than women and occasionally will develop a diffuse sebaceous enlargement of the entire nose, thus giving the face a distorted appearance.

RECOMMENDED TREATMENT

Seborrhea can adequately be treated by washing the face as frequently as possible and shampooing the hair regularly. Alcohol pads may be carried during the day, so that excessive grease and oil can be quickly removed at any time with just a gentle swabbing.

For seborrheic dermatitis, more aggressive therapy is needed. At first, sulfur and salicylic acid creams and lotions should be tried. These will break up and dissolve large scales and aid in their removal from the skin. For problem cases, or when salicylic acid and sulfur are insufficient, coal tar derivatives must be used. For additional comments on the above medications, refer to Chapter 12, "Dandruff" (pages 146-47).

COMMENTS AND CAUTIONS

If superficial bacterial infections complicate the course of seborrhea, topical antibiotics should be used. For information about these products, see Chapter 11, "Cuts, Scrapes, and Scratches" (page 142).

For difficult or extensive cases, treatment must be directed by a physician, and prescription products may be needed.

SEBORRHEA MEDICATIONS

For a listing of these medications, please turn to Chapter 12, "Dandruff" (pages 147-51).

32. Sprains and Strains
(Muscular and joint aches and pains)

The expression "muscular aches and pains" is self-explanatory, but why do they occur?
Muscular aches and pains are experienced by everyone in all walks of life. People who get little exercise will develop muscle soreness twelve to twenty-four hours after moderate physical exertion. Laborers, who must use their bodies every day, can also experience soreness and stiffness after an exceptionally laborious job or following muscle injury. Furthermore, diffuse muscular aches and pains frequently accompany colds and flus. These ailments are common and fairly well recognized.

Other more serious causes of muscular pain include muscle ruptures or tears, bruises with internal bleeding, and even tumor growths within the muscle. However, these conditions can usually be distinguished from the more common, less significant causes of muscular pain, because accompanying symptoms—such as muscle swelling, discoloration, and severe pain—result with ruptures or deep extensive bruises; and a hard, slow-growing nodule within the muscle is usually an obvious sign of tumor growth.

Why do joint pains occur?
Joint pains occur for many reasons, but the more common causes include arthritis, bursitis, and tendinitis.

Tendinitis generally follows physical exertion (tennis for example), in which the fibrous connections between the muscles and bones are stretched excessively and thus receive minor damage or destruction. Pain will occur quickly, but it will gradually disappear as long as continued insult does not take place. Degeneration of the tendon will occur if frequent injury is sustained.

Bursitis is an inflammation of the fibrous tissue sac (bursa) that surrounds the joints of the body. It may be caused by trauma, infection, or other medical problems like gout and arthritis. When inflamed, the bursae become swollen, irritated, and painful.

Arthritis, like bursitis, is an inflammation of the joints, but, in this condition, the site of injury is the joint's surface where one bone moves against another, rather than the fibrous sac that surrounds each joint. Arthritis, bursitis, and tendinitis all result in tenderness or pain at the joint, limitation of movement, and variable swelling. Arthritis is usually worse following long periods of inactivity and upon arising in the morning. Tendinitis is worse following exercise.

What can be done for muscle and joint aches and pains?
Specific treatment depends on the exact nature of the illness. Persistent conditions, such as rheumatoid arthritis, should be directed to the attention of a physician. However, temporary relief for all the conditions, which is all that is necessary in many cases, can be achieved in several different ways.

Local heat can be applied to the affected muscle or joint by way of a heating pad or warm-water soaks. Not only will this therapy provide soothing relief, it will also promote local repair of injured tissues and rapid healing. Damp heat, which is more penetrating than dry heat, is preferable.

Minor pain relievers, such as aspirin and acetaminophen, will be of great benefit for the discomfort of joint and muscle injuries and will work effectively for the aches and pains associated with colds and flus as well.

A host of topical liniments and creams, which are massaged into the painful muscles or joints, also have a beneficial, although limited, effect and can be used safely in a great majority of cases. These preparations, however, should never be used while dry or wet heat is being applied simultaneously to the same areas of soreness.

In addition to the above treatments, immediate immobilization of the injured muscles or joints will aid in early healing, but motion should be resumed as soon as possible in order to prevent joints from becoming stiff and permanently disabled.

What are the ingredients of the topical ointments, lotions, and liniments, and how do they work?

Allyl isothiocyanate, camphor, capsicum, clove oil, menthol, methyl salicylate, thymol, and turpentine oil are combined or used separately as topical pain relievers. Their exact mode of action is poorly understood and, without a doubt, much of their effect is psychological. However, their benefit is well recognized by the millions of people who use them.

Possibly these substances increase the supply of blood reaching the painful muscle or joint by a reflex nerve action. Maybe they are absorbed through the skin and actually reach the affected area, thus bringing the minor anesthetic qualities they possess directly to the point of irritation. Although these theories are only speculative, the pain relief seems real enough to warrant the select and limited use of these agents.

RECOMMENDED TREATMENT

It is truly difficult to evaluate these products, especially since most of them contain the same ingredients and comparative studies are unavailable. I suggest one that incorporates methyl salicylate, menthol, and camphor.

COMMENTS AND CAUTIONS

The vast majority of muscular and joint pains are transient and pass quickly. Self-treatment is all that is needed to care for these problems. Other times, however, the ailments are better treated by a physician. If your condition is associated with a fever, rash, inability to move the joint, a lump in a muscle, or severe pain and swelling see your doctor. If problems that at first seemed minor persist for more than a month or worsen, a doctor's examination is also indicated.

EXTERNAL ANALGESICS
Boldface: Recommended

Absorbent Rub, lotion	methyl salicylate 0.7% camphor 1.6% menthol 1.6% wormwood oil 0.6% sassafras oil 0.5% capsicum 0.03% isopropyl alcohol 69% green soap 11.6% pine tar soap 0.9% o-phenylphcnol 0.5% benzocaine 0.5%
Absorbine Arthritic, lotion	methyl salicylate menthol methyl nicotinate emulsion base
Absorbine Jr., lotion	wormwood oil thymol menthol chloroxylenol acetone
Act-on Rub, lotion	methyl salicylate menthol camphor eucalyptus oil mustard oil isopropyl myristate balm base lanolin
Analbalm, lotion	methyl salicylate 5% menthol 0.5% camphor 2.5% emulsion base

Analgesic Balm, ointment	methyl salicylate 15% menthol 15% hydrocarbon waxes lanolin petrolatum sorbitan sesquioleate water base
Analgesic Balm, ointment	methyl salicylate 15% menthol 15%
Antiphlogistine, poultice	methyl salicylate eucalyptus oil salicylic acid glycerin kaolin boric acid peppermint oil
Arthralgen, ointment	methyl salicylate 15% menthol 10% thymol 1% methacholine chloride 0.25%
Banalg, lotion	methyl salicylate menthol camphor eucalyptus oil greaseless base
Baumodyne, gel	menthol
Ben-Gay, lotion	methyl salicylate 15% menthol 10% greaseless base
Braska, lotion	methyl salicylate menthol camphor monoglycol salicylate methyl nicotinate salicylamide isopropyl alcohol
Chloro-Salicylate, ointment	methyl salicylate 6.66 g/30 g menthol 1.134 g/30 g chloral hydrate 648 mg/30 g

Counterpain Rub,
ointment

methyl salicylate 10.2%
menthol 5.4%
eugenol 1.4%

Dencorub, lotion

methyl salicylate
menthol
camphor

Emul-O-Balm,
lotion

methyl salicylate 22.45 mg/1 ml
menthol 22.45 mg/1 ml
camphor 11.22 mg/1 ml
ribbon gum tragacanth 8.37 mg/1 ml
methylparaben 1.50 mg/1 ml
propylparaben 0.30 mg/1 ml

End-Ake, liniment

methyl salicylate
menthol
camphor
eucalyptus oil

Exocaine Plus,
ointment

methyl salicylate 30%
menthol crystals 2%
clove oil 1%
benzocaine 5%

Exocaine Tube,
ointment

methyl salicylate 30%
clove oil 1%
benzocaine 5%

Girofoam, aerosol
foam

methyl salicylate 30%
benzocaine 3%
volatile oils

Go-Pain, balm/
lotion

methyl nicotinate
methyl salicylate
menthol
camphor

Heet, lotion

methyl salicylate
camphor
capsicum
alcohol 53%

Heet, spray	methyl salicylate 25% menthol 3% camphor 1.5% methyl nicotinate 1% alcohol 29.5%
Icy Hot, liniment	methyl salicylate menthol
Infra-Rub, cream	methyl nicotinate histamine dihydrochloride capsicum oleoresin glycol monosalicylate
Lini Balm, aerosol foam	methyl salicylate 15% menthol 1% camphor 2% eucalyptus oil 2% polyoxyalkalene lanolin
Mentholatum, ointment	menthol 1.35% camphor 9% aromatic oils petrolatum
Mentholatum Deep Heating, ointment	methyl salicylate 12.7% menthol 6% eucalyptus oil turpentine oil lanolin greaseless base
Mentholatum Deep Heating, lotion	methyl salicylate 12.7% menthol 6% lanolin greaseless base
Minit-Rub, ointment	methyl salicylate 10% menthol 3.54% camphor 4.44% eucalyptus oil 1.77% anhydrous lanolin 4.44%
Mobisyl, cream	triethylanolamine salicylate 20%

**Musterole Deep
Strength, ointment**

methyl salicylate 30%
menthol 3%
methyl nicotinate 0.5%

Musterole Regular
or Extra Strength,
ointment

methyl salicylate
menthol
camphor
mustard oil
glycol monosalicylate

Musterole Children's
Strength, ointment

methyl salicylate
menthol
camphor
glycol monosalicylate

Neurabalm, lotion

methyl salicylate
menthol
camphor
eucalyptus oil
cajuput oil
chlorothymol
alcohol 54%
acetone
benzocaine

Omega Oil, lotion

methyl salicylate
methyl nicotinate
capsicum oleoresin
histamine dihydrochloride
isopropyl alcohol 44.4%

**Panalgesic, lotion,
spray**

methyl salicylate 50%
menthol 2%
camphor 4%
emollient oils 20%
alcohol 18%
aspirin 8%

Penetro Quick
Acting Rub,
ointment

methyl salicylate
menthol
camphor
turpentine
thymol
pine oil

Sloan's, liniment

methyl salicylate 2.66%
camphor 3.35%
turpentine oil 46.76%
pine oil 6.74%
capsicum oleoresin 0.62%
kerosene 29.88%

Soltice Hi-Therm, cream

methyl salicylate 50 mg/1 g
menthol 70 mg/1 g
camphor 50 mg/1 g
eucalyptus oil 10 mg/1 g
greaseless base

Soltice Quick Rub, cream

methyl salicylate 50 mg/1 g
menthol 50 mg/1 g
camphor 50 mg/1 g
eucalyptus oil 10 mg/1 g
greaseless base

SPD, lotion

methyl salicylate 10%
menthol
camphor
methyl nicotinate 1%
washable greaseless base

SPD, cream

methyl salicylate 10%
menthol
camphor
methyl nicotinate 1%
capsicum oleoresin 0.5%
washable greaseless base

Stimurub, ointment

methyl salicylate
menthol
capsicum oleoresin

Surin, ointment

methyl salicylate
menthol
camphor
methacholine chloride 0.25%
greaseless base

Vicks Vaporub,
external rub

menthol
camphor
turpentine spirits
eucalyptus oil
cedar leaf oil
myristica oil
thymol

Yager's, liniment

camphor 1%
turpentine oil 8%
aqua ammonia 1.4%
ammonium oleate

Zemo Liquid, lotion

methyl salicylate
menthol
thymol
eucalyptol
phenol
sodium salicylate
sodium borate
benzoic acid
boric acid
alcohol 35%

Zemo Liquid Extra
Strength, lotion

methyl salidylate
menthol
thymol
eucalyptol
phenol
sodium salicylate
sodium borate
benzoic acid
boric acid
alcohol

33. Sunburn

What is a sunburn?
A sunburn is the result of overexposure to sunlight which causes heat and light damage to the skin.

What changes occur with sunburns
The most obvious change is a reddening of the skin that varies in intensity, depending on the amount of time spent in the sun, sometimes occurring after only twenty minutes exposure. The redness is caused by an increase in the amount of blood that is present in the millions of tiny blood vessels in the exposed skin.

A second change that might be noted in more severe cases is swelling of the skin caused by damage to the blood vessels which results in leaking fluids collecting in the skin. Water blisters may even develop.

Is sunburn damage reversible?
Yes, for the most part, the skin damage associated with sunburns is reversible. Mild sunburns usually disappear within several days, but severe sunburns may actually take weeks to heal and then leave destructive changes in blood vessels that may be present for many months. If a person is foolish enough to sunburn frequently, skin changes that are not reversible will often result. The elastic fibers in the dermis eventually become totally degenerated, leaving the skin "old" and wrinkled. Blotching and thickening occasionally develop. These changes will especially occur to

320

those who are occupationally open to continuous sun exposure, such as farmers and fishermen.

Can the destruction of sunburn be prevented?
Certainly. Avoiding excessive sun exposure is a sure way to prevent sunburn and to reduce sun damage to the skin. Blonds and redheads, young children and babies, and all those people with sun sensitivity are wise to follow this procedure. In addition, sunscreens also help and should be used whenever a day in the sun is anticipated.

What are sunscreens?
As the name indicates, sunscreens are preparations that shield the skin from the sun. When used as directed, they help to prevent sunburn by blocking out harmful ultraviolet light.

How do sunscreens work?
There are two general types of sunscreens. Sunscreens that are physically active work by setting up a barrier which will not let ultraviolet light reach the skin. Zinc oxide, a thick white paste, protects in this manner. Sunscreens that are chemically active provide skin protection by actually absorbing ultraviolet light and converting it to another form of energy, such as heat or fluorescence.

What qualities are desirable in a sunscreen?
An effective sunscreen should have the following qualities:
1. Broad-range; blocks out or absorbs all harmful rays.
2. Nonirritating; can be used regularly and frequently.
3. Stability; does not decompose or break down easily.
4. Long-lasting; remains on the skin in an adequate layer.

Who should use sunscreen products?
In my opinion, anyone who receives prolonged sun exposure should use these products. This particularly includes the "sun whorshippers," those people who desire a rich tan and sunbathe frequently, and also those people who work contin-

uously outdoors. Obviously children, and also adults, with fair skin should protect themselves whenever they anticipate a full day in the sun. First day sunbathers can prevent that "first day sunburn" with sunscreen products.

Do sunscreens only prevent sunburn?
No. Sunscreens will also reduce the harmful, aginglike effects that can be caused by the sun. When used continuously and started at an early age, sunscreen products will help maintain a vibrant, more youthful appearing skin.

There are other situations where the use of sunscreens proves helpful. Certain individuals suffer from allergic reactions to sunlight. Some of these allergic reactions are related to specific drug therapy and are characterized by a sunburnlike condition that occurs after only short exposure. Specific drugs known to cause photosensitivity reactions include chlorothiazide, tetracyclines, sulfa drugs, barbiturates, erythromycin, chlorpromazine, and minor tranquilizers. If you are taking any drug and become overly sensitive to sunlight, consult your doctor about possible changing medicines. If changing drugs is impossible, sunscreens should be used whenever you spend any time outdoors.

Since many forms of skin cancer are related to sun exposure, can the use of sunscreens reduce this hazard?
Absolutely! Many studies have shown a direct relationship between sun exposure and skin cancer, actinic dermatitis, and other major skin disorders. People who live in the sun belt bear a much greater risk of developing skin cancer than their northern counterparts. This is especially true of fair-skinned people and those who must work outside. The regular use of a sunscreen can significantly reduce the possibility of developing any sun-related skin disorder, including skin cancer.

Will sunscreens prevent tanning?
Not necessarily. Since the light rays that cause sunburns also promote tanning, sunscreens will block both effects. However, a tan can still be obtained if the sunscreen is used

less frequently than recommended or in lesser amounts. For those individuals who generally tan rather than burn, the use of a sunscreen on those areas of the body that are greatly exposed—the nose, forehead, cheeks—will provide more even tanning and less cracking and peeling.

Since herpes simplex eruptions are associated with sun exposure, will sunscreens prevent their occurrence?
Herpes simplex is a specific type of virus that is associated with many illnesses, including the common fever blister, which is a small sensitive sore or eruption that breaks out on the lips. Many people notice that these eruptions develop after a day in the sun, and it has been established that sunlight can, indeed, activate the herpes virus. Since sunscreens block out sunlight, their application to the lips prior to sun exposure can significantly prevent fever blister recurrences.

If sunscreens are not employed and long days are spent in the sun, what is the result?
The result is usually sunburn and the symptoms that accompany this senseless disorder.

In a mild case, local heat or a slight burning sensation is noted over exposed areas of the body. More severe burns may be followed by skin swelling, blisters, and great physical discomfort. Contact with clothing or any other material may be unbearable. And when sunburns are extreme, chills, fever, nausea, and vomiting may take place. Shock may even occur.

What can be done for sunburns?
When sunburns are severe or extreme, a doctor should be sought, especially if shock is suspected. Mild to moderate sunburns can be self-treated easily with rest, soothing lotions, cool water baths, and oral fluids.

What soothing lotions can be used to aid sunburn victims?

The most popular lotions or sprays available for sunburn relief are those that contain a local anesthetic, which is a substance that temporarily deadens nerves and prevents the sensation of pain. Although they have no healing effect on the skin, local anesthetics do provide some relief for the sunburn sufferer.

The majority of products available over the counter contain benzocaine combined with several other ingredients that have a variety of purposes. Lidocaine, dibucaine, tetracaine, ethyl chloride, butamben picrate, phenylphenol, and diperodon are other local anesthetics which are found in sunburn preparations, but, by far, benzocaine is the most popular.

Do these products really work?

For any medication to be effective, it must be used in adequate concentrations, and herein lies the problem with most sunburn pain relievers: they just aren't strong enough. Benzocaine, for example, must be used in concentrations of about 20 percent in order to penetrate the skin, numb superficial nerves, and block pain.

Are there any OTC sunburn products that have sufficient amounts of pain-relieving ingredients?

Yes, but they are few in number and have common, and sometimes significant, side effects.

RECOMMENDED TREATMENT

I think that most minor to moderate sunburns should be left alone. A cool water, soapless bath may be sufficiently soothing to help you through the initial crisis. If possible, sunburn products which contain local anesthetics should be used as infrequently as possible because sensitivities to these products have been reported. However, when physical discomfort is extreme, benzocaine in 20 percent solutions should help.

Insofar as selecting an effective sunscreen is concerned, several independent studies have shown 5 percent para-aminobenzoic acid to be a very effective sunscreen which is well tolerated by almost everyone. It demonstrates great absorbing quality for ultraviolet light and has been highly recommended in the past. Twenty percent isoamyl NN dimethylaminobenzoate receives equal praise. Also useful as general sunscreens, but particularly effective in preventing sun sensitivity, are 3 percent dioxybenzone, 3 percent oxybenzone, and 10 percent sulisobenzone.

Although 5 percent para-aminobenzoic acid is considered to be the best all-around sunscreen, it does have one drawback. In certain individuals, it produces a red irritation of the skin. If you use a sunscreen that contains this compound, remember its possible irritating potential and switch to another product that contains oxybenzone, dioxybenzone, or sulisobenzone if reddening develops. These should work equally well without the irritating side effect.

COMMENTS AND CAUTIONS

I don't have to tell you how common sunburns are or how quickly they can develop when we spend those wonderful sunny days outdoors. But I will tell you this. Sunburns can be very serious ailments and should be prevented. Prevention is easily accomplished using one of the sunscreen products discussed in this chapter.

If you develop a sunburn, follow the instructions I have given you; however, when the sunburn is associated with light-headedness, dizziness, nausea, vomiting, or fainting, call your doctor or emergency service. Sunburned infants should likewise be seen by a doctor.

A word about tanning. There are many sunscreens and suntanning products on the market, so it is quite easy to become confused or misled. I personally have seen people burn to a crisp on the beach because they failed to use an adequate product or were so foolish that they used no product at all. Sun-sensitive and fair-skinned individuals should always use sunscreens, and this applies to babies and young children as well. Those who will tan normally should initially use sunscreens their first few days in the sun. Then, after a base tan has been obtained, a suntan lotion may be used, aided by a sunscreen to protect those overly exposed areas such as the forehead, nose, and cheeks.

I highly discourage the use of oils, butters, gels, and greases which contain no active sunscreen compounds, because these products actually promote burning. People who use them on their first big day in the sun will probably spend the next day in bed. And, those people with good tans, who only use oils, will probably stay dark, but in time they will notice destructive skin changes caused by the sun.

SUNBURN MEDICATION

SUNBURN RELIEF REMEDIES
Boldface: Recommended

Aerosept, aerosol	lidocaine cetyltrimethylammonium bromide chloroxylenol fragrance
Americaine, aerosol	benzocaine 20% water base
Americaine, ointment	benzocaine 20% benzethonium chloride 0.1% polyethylene glycols
Bactine, liquid	methylbenzethonium chloride 0.5% chlorothymol 0.1% alcohol 3.17% tyloxapol 0.35%
Betadine, aerosol	povidone-iodine 5% water base

Betadine, ointment   povidone-iodine 10%
                     water base

Burn-A-Lay, cream   benzocaine 1.25%
                     chlorobutanol 0.75%
                     benzoxyquine 0.025%
                     zinc oxide 2%
                     thymol 0.5%

Burn Relief Spray   benzocaine
                     chlorobutanol 0.3%
                     benzethonium chloride
                     polyalkylene glycol
                     menthol
                     isopropyl alcohol 11%

Burntame Spray   benzocaine 20%
                     8-hydroxyquinoline

Butesin Picrate,   butamben picrate 1%
ointment

Dermoplast, spray   benzocaine 4.5%
                     benzethonium chloride 0.1%
                     methylparaben 2%
                     isopropyl alcohol 1.9%
                     menthol 0.5%

Foille, aerosol   benzocaine 2%
                     benzyl alcohol 4%
                     8-hydroxyquinoline
                     sulfur
                     oil

Foille, liquid   benzocaine 2%
                     benzyl alcohol 4%
                     8-hydroxyquinoline
                     sulfur
                     oil

Foille, ointment   benzocaine 2%
                     benzyl alcohol 4%
                     8-hydroxyquinoline
                     sulfur
                     oil

Gebauer's Tannic Spray	benzocaine 0.5% ethyl chloride 33.3% chlorobutanol 1.2% tannic acid 3.9% menthol 0.1%
Hist-A-Balm Medicated Lotion	diperodon hydrochloride 0.25% benzalkonium chloride 0.1% phenyltoloxamine dihydrogen citrate 0.75% menthol camphor
Hyrocain, cream	benzocaine dibucaine tetracaine
Kip First Aid Spray, aerosol	benzocaine 3% o-phenylphenol 0.5% oils methyl salicylate salicylic acid
Kip First Aid Spray, lotion	benzocaine 3% o-phenylphenol 0.5% oils methyl salicylate salicylic acid
Kip for Burns, ointment	o-phenylphenol 0.5% phenol 0.5% oils methyl salicylate salicylic acid zinc oxide petrolatum paraffin lanolin
Kip Moisturizing Lotion	benzocaine 2% benzalkonium chloride salicylic acid stearic acid glyceryl monostearate oils

isopropyl myristate
propylene glycol
triethanolamine
methylparaben
butylated hydroxyanisole
fragrance

Kip Sunburn Spray,
aerosol

benzocaine 10%
benzalkonium chloride
menthol
lanolin
propylene glycol
isopropyl alcohol 7%
hexadecyl alcohol

Medicone Dressing
Cream

benzocaine 5 mg/1 g
8-hydroxyquinoline sulfate 0.5 mg/1 g
cod liver oil 125 mg/1 g
zinc oxide 125 mg/1 g
menthol 1.8 mg/1 g
petrolatum
lanolin
paraffin
talc
fragrance

Mediconet, wipes

benzalkonium chloride 0.02%
hamamelis water 50%
glycerin 10
lanolin 0.5%
methylparaben 0.15%
fragrance

Medi-Quik, aerosol

lidocaine
benzalkonium chloride
isopropyl alcohol 12%

Medi-Quik, pump
spray

lidocaine
benzalkonium chloride
isopropyl alcohol 79%

Morusan, ointment

benzocaine 2%
cod liver oil concentrate
lanolin
petrolatum

Noxema Medicated, cream	phenol, less than 0.5% menthol camphor oils lime water water base
Noxema Medicated, lotion	phenol, less than 0.5% menthol camphor oils lime water water base
Noxema Sunburn Spray, aerosol	benzocaine 1% benzalkonium chloride 0.1% menthol 0.1% alcohol 7% emollient
Nupercainal Cream	dibucaine 0.5% acetone sodium bisulfite 0.37% water base
Nupercainal Ointment	dibucaine 1% acetone sodium bisulfite 0.5%
Nupercainal Spray	dibucaine 0.25% alcohol 46%
Obtundia Cream	cresol-camphor complex
Panthoderm Cream	dexpanthenol 2% water base
Pontocaine, cream	tetracaine 1% water base
Pontocaine, ointment	tetracaine 0.5% menthol 0.5% white petrolatum white wax

Rexall First Aid benzocaine
Spray chlorothymol
methylbenzethonium chloride
isopropyl alcohol 4%
tyloxapol
camphor

Solarcaine Cream benzocaine 1%
triclosan
menthol
camphor

Solarcaine Foam benzocaine 0.5%
triclosan
menthol
camphor

Solarcaine Lotion benzocaine 0.5%
triclosan
menthol
camphor

Solarcaine Spray benzocaine 5%
triclosan

Tanurol, ointment benzocaine 1%
tannic acid 3%
phenol 0.75%

Tega Caine, aerosol benzocaine 20%
benzyl alcohol 2.3%
chloroxylenol 0.51%
urea 5.38%
propylene glycol

Unburn, cream, benzocaine
lotion o-phenylphenol
menthol
lanolin
water base

Unburn Spray benzocaine
chloroxylenol
menthol
lanolin
alcohol 7%

Unguentine, aerosol spray	benzocaine benzalkonium chloride chloroxylenol menthol alcohol 7%
Unguentine, cream	parahydracin benzalkonium chloride phenyl 1% aluminum hydroxide zinc carbonate zinc acetate zinc oxide oils menthol eugenol
Unguentine Plus, cream	lidocaine chloroxylenol aluminum hydroxide zinc carbonate zinc acetate zinc oxide phenol oils menthol eugenol
Utesin Picrate, ointment	butamben picrate 1%
Vaseline Pure Petroleum Jelly	white petrolatum 100%
Xylocaine, ointment	lidocaine 2.5% polyethylene glycols propylene glycol

SUNSCREEN PRODUCTS

A-Fil Cream	menthyl anthranilate 5% titanium dioxide 5%
Block Out, liquid	padimate 3.6% alcohol 70%

	moisturizers fragrance
Coppertone Nosekote, liquid	homosalate 7%
Coppertone Shade Lotion	homosalate 5% padimate 2%
Coppertone Suntan Foam	homosalate 8%
Coppertone Suntan Lotion	homosalate 8%
Coppertone Suntan Oil	homosalate 9%
Coppertone Suntan Spray	homosalate 9%
Coppertone Tanning Butter Cream	homosalate 8%
Coppertone Tanning Butter Spray	homosalate 8%
Dark Tanning Oil	padimate 1.1% mineral oil emollients moisturizers
Eclipse, lotion	glyceryl p-aminobenzoate 3% padimate 3% alcohol 5% oleth-3 phosphate petrolatum synthetic spermaceti glycerin mineral oil lanolin alcohol cetyl stearyl glycol lanolin oil triethanolamine carbomer 934P benzyl alcohol 0.5% fragrance

Florida Tan Tanning Oil And Dark Tanning Oil	aminobenzoic acid cocoa butter coconut oil aloe almond oil lanolin banana fragrance
Golden Tan Lotion	padimate 1% cocoa butter mineral oil lanolin alcohol
Indoor/Outdoor Foam	padimate 1.05% dihydroxyacetone 4% lanolin glycerin mineral oil
Indoor/Outdoor Lotion	padimate 1.05% dihydroxyacetone 4% lanolin mineral oil
Maxafil Cream	menthyl anthranilate 5% cinoxate 4%
Mentholatum Stick	padimate petrolatum menthol camphor oils
Natural Woman Suntan Lotion	oxybenzone dioxybenzone
Pabafilm, liquid	isoamyl NN dimethylaminobenzoate 2.5% alcohol 70%
Pabagel, gel	aminobenzoic acid 5% alcohol 57%
Pabanol, liquid	aminobenzoic acid 5% alcohol 70%

Paba Sun Lotion	aminobenzoic acid allantoin cocoa butter vitamins A, D, E sesame oil avocado oil
Presun, liquid	p-amino benzoic acid 5% alcohol 55%
Q.T. Quick Tanning Foam	homosalate 8% dihydroxyacetone
Q.T. Quick Tanning Lotion	homosalate 8% dihydroxyacetone
RVPaba Stick	aminobenzoic acid red petrolatum
RVPaque, ointment	cinoxate red petrolatum zinc oxide
Sea & Ski Lotion	glyceryl p-aminobenzoate 2% glycerin mineral oil lanolin sesame oil
Smootie, lotion	padimate 2.5% glycerin stearic acid dimethicone
Solar Cream	aminobenzoic acid 4% titanium dioxide 12% cream base 84%
Solbar, lotion	dioxybenzone 3% oxybenzone 3%
Sudden Tan Foam	homosalate 6.25% dihydroxyacetone
Sudden Tan Lotion	homosalate 6.25% dihydroxyacetone

Sundare Clear, lotion	cinoxate 1.75% alcohol 51.8%
Sundare Creamy, lotion	cinoxate 2% lanolin derivative
Sungard, lotion	sulisobenzone 10%
Sunswept, cream	digalloyl trioleate 3.5%
Super Shade Lotion	aminobenzoic acid 5%
Swedish Tanning Secret Lotion	padimate 1.5% emollient
Swedish Tanning Secret Oil	padimate 1.2% oil
Tega-Tan Foam	glyceryl p-aminobenzoate emulsifier alcohol fragrance
Tropic Sun Oil	padimate 1.1% cocoa butter coconut oil almond oil mineral oil lanolin
Uval Sun 'N Wind Stick	padimate 3%
Uval Sunscreen Lotion	sulisobenzone 10%

34. Warts

Exactly what are warts?
Warts are small, raised skin growths that are caused by the smallest of living organisms, the virus, from the papovavirus group.

How do warts develop?
Warts develop like any other superficial infection. First, the virus must come in contact with the skin, and this may follow a simple handshake. Then extension through the surface layer of dead skin cells must take place. For this to happen, a small break or tear in the skin must exist, allowing the virus free access to deeper, living cells which can then be infected.

Once inside the viable cells, the virus can multiply and flourish, using the host's cellular nutrients for sustenance. During the period of infection, the virus also stimulates the infected skin cells to grow and divide, producing the small warty lesions that you soon notice.

Who is affected?
Anyone, old or young, male or female, can develop warts. However, they are most common in older children and adults under thirty.

Where do warts commonly appear?
Warts develop on various areas of the body and are named according to location or appearance.

For instance, plantar warts grow on the plantar, bottom,

surface of the feet and may become flattened by the pressure of walking.

Genital warts arise on the head and shaft of the penis or on the vulva, vagina, or cervix. These sexually transmitted warts may also occur in or around the anus. They are pink to tan and have a cauliflowerlike appearance.

Juvenile, flattop warts are usually small and are predominantly found in clusters on the face and neck or along the wrists and hands.

Filiform warts are usually long and narrow as the name implies. They generally grow about the face, commonly on the eyelids and lips, but also occur on the neck.

Common warts, the ones most easily recognized, develop on the hands and fingers.

What is the expected course of a wart?

Although 50 percent of the warts you notice will disappear without any treatment, others spread and sprout abundantly, seeded by the virus of the original lesion. Scratching and picking at the mother wart not only promotes expansion to new areas by surfacing the existing viruses but also stimulates the manipulated mother wart to enlarge and thicken.

About 30 percent of warts that are surgically or chemically removed will regrow.

How can warts be removed?

Surgically removing warts involves cutting them off, burning them away, or freezing them. Each of these modes requires professional techniques. Other methods of wart removal include chemical dissolution or physical scrapping, which can be accomplished at home with the use of OTC products.

What are the ingredients in OTC chemical wart removers, and do they really work?

There are four basic kinds of medications that are incorporated in OTC wart-removing products.

Ascorbic acid: Ascorbic acid, vitamin C, is necessary for

normal tissue growth and repair but has no established role in the removal of warts.

Castor oil: Castor oil might soften a wart and allow deeper penetration of acceptable wart-removing compounds but has no intrinsic antiwart value itself.

Benzoic acid, glacial acetic acid, lactic acid, salicylic acid, pantothenic acid, phenoxyethanoic acid: Each of these acids effectively destroys warts by caustically disrupting and digesting the lesion and the virus. They will also eat through normal healthy skin and must therefore be used with caution.

Of the six, glacial acetic acid and lactic acid are the most corrosive and are used in 10 to 20 percent solutions. Salicylic acid must be present in higher concentrations, 20 to 40 percent, when used separately but may be present in 15 percent solutions when combined with other acids. Five percent pantothenic acid is also effective.

Zinc chloride: Another caustic compound, zinc chloride, will also remove warts through its corrosive effect on the skin and is used in relatively low concentrations, 1 to 3 percent.

RECOMMENDED TREATMENT
Products which contain any of the previously mentioned acids, either alone or in combination, in the appropriate concentrations can be used effectively if applied properly. At times, wart removal is a slow process, so therapy must be prolonged to be effective.

COMMENTS AND CAUTIONS
As previously mentioned, the wart removers are very corrosive substances. They will destroy normal skin and can seriously damage the eyes and other sensitive tissues. If they are used, care must be taken to cover the wart only, not the surrounding skin. I do not think they should be used on the face or on large clusters of warts anywhere else on the body.

Other restrictions also exist. If you are diabetic or suffer from poor circulation, these products are not for you. Their use is also discouraged if bleeding or infection develops at the site of application.

For venereal warts, treatment by a physician is advised because of the corrosive nature of the wart-removing compounds and the possibility of permanent scarring that is inherent in each of these products.

WART REMOVERS

Boldface: Recommended

Bevill's Corn Remedy	salicylic acid ferric chloride tincture alcohol ether methyl salicylate
Blis-to-Sol Corn And Callus Remover	salicylic acid 18% diperodon hydrochloride 1% zinc chloride
Blue Jay Callus Pads and Discs	phenoxyethanoic acid
Blue Jay Callus Plaster	phenoxyethanoic acid
Blue Jay Pads	phenoxyethanoic acid
Blue Jay Corn Pads	phenoxyethanoic acid
Blue Jay Corn Pad Treatment	phenoxyethanoic acid benzocaine chlorobutanol thymol benzoxyquine zinc oxide
Blue Jay Corn Plaster	phenoxyethanoic acid

Blue Jay Liquid Corn-Callus Remover	phenoxyethanoic acid pyroxylin acetone
Compound W Wart Remover	salicylic acid 14% glacial acetic acid 11% menthol 2% camphor 1.5% castor oil alcohol ether acetone
Derma-Soft Creme	salicylic acid 2.5%
Dr. Scholl's Corn/ Callous Salve	salicylic acid eucalyptus oil petrolatum lanolin mineral oil
Dr. Scholl's "2" Drop Corn-Callous Remover	salicylic acid camphor alcohol 15% ether
Dr. Scholl's Fixo Corn Plaster	salicylic acid
Dr. Scholl's Waterproof Corn Pads	salicylic acid
Dr. Scholl's Zino- Pads	salicylic acid
Freezone Corn and Callus Remover	salicylic acid zinc chloride 8.75 g/oz alcohol 20.8% ether castor oil
Solvex, liquid	salicylic acid benzoic acid benzocaine chlorothymol alcohol 45%

Vergo, ointment   calcium pantothenate
          ascorbic acid

Wartaway, liquid   salicylic acid
          glacial acetic acid
          camphor
          castor oil

Wart Fix, liquid   castor oil

Afterword

ADVICE TO THE TRAVELER

Traveling can be the best experience of your life, or it can be the worst—if you get sick, that is. Here are some helpful suggestions to better prepare yourself for the common ailments of traveling.

What shots will you need?
Immunization requirements are constantly changing and relate to diseases that are common in different parts of the world. You can determine which shots you will need by calling your local health department or travel agent. Either of these groups should be able to describe the specific diseases you might encounter in your travels and relate information that might help you avoid them.

Here are a few important things to remember.

1. Begin inoculations two months in advance.

2. Receive all *required* shots and also all *recommended* shots.

3. Record all immunizations in the International Certificate of Vaccination book, issued by the U.S. Public Health Service. (This is extremely important because if the shots are not recorded properly, they will not be accepted and you will have to be reimmunized.)

What about the water?
In less sophisticated countries, water can be a problem, but only if you let it. When in doubt about tap water quality, don't drink it. Bottled water, beer, and wine are usually safe and can easily be substituted for tap water. Be sure to insist

that the bottles are opened at your table to help insure that the contents are original and not locally rebottled with contaminated fluid.

When questionable water must be consumed because substitutes are unavailable, purify it yourself with halazone tablets or by boiling.

And remember: Swimming in pools, lakes, streams, and rivers usually leads to swallowing some water which might be an overlooked means of contamination and illness.

What about milk?
In many underdeveloped countries, milk should also be avoided because it transmits tuberculosis and brucellosis. Improper bottling may further introduce other forms of bacteria and contribute to a variety of illnesses. If milk must be consumed, boil it first.

What foods should you eat?
In developed countries, food will rarely cause illness except for possible indigestion from overeating. Simply apply the principles of good eating habits wherever you go.

In underdeveloped countries, where food can be a problem, make sure meat, fish, and poultry are cooked properly. Always wash raw fruit and vegetables before eating them. And, avoid poorly processed and poorly stored foods such as cold platters, previously prepared dishes, and salads.

If you should find yourself in a dilemma, as long as the food is thoroughly cooked and served piping hot, don't worry.

Regardless of where you dine, always wash your hands before eating.

Are eating utensils safe
Usually eating utensils present no problem, but if you notice improperly cleaned silverware or plates, have them rewashed. If this is impossible, wipe them yourself with a clean napkin or a prepackaged moistened towel that you can carry with you.

If you become ill while traveling, what can you do?
If the problem is minor and you have prepared yourself in advance by applying the principles discussed in this chapter, treat yourself. Many times physicians in out-of-the-way places or undeveloped nations are poorly qualified and may cause additional problems and suffering. Only consult them when absolutely necessary.

Doctors in all of the developed countries are generally well trained and competent.

How can you find a doctor while traveling?
By calling the American Embassy wherever you may be, good medical advice can be obtained. A list of physicians and surgeons is always kept on hand and constantly updated for your convenience. Additional advice is available through local airlines, travel bureaus, and shipping lines. And if all else fails, contact any available American or European missionary service; trained medical personnel usually travel with these groups.

In advance of travel, you can write to InterMedic, 777 Third Avenue, New York, N.Y. 10017, or the International Association for Medical Assistance to Travelers for the names and addresses of physicians in the countries you intend to visit.

What medications should you take?
If you suffer from a particular ailment that requires prescription drugs, take an ample supply with you and also take an extra prescription for a new supply, just to be safe.

In lieu of any particular problems, the list of products at the end of the chapter should take care of most common traveling ailments.

If a simple unexpected ailment develops and you have no medication on hand, what should you do?
This can be a problem, but don't despair. Frequently, the exact same products that are found in the United States are

exported to foreign countries. Although they may cost a little more, they'll be worth every penny. Buy them!

What happens if you can't find any recognizable products?
When American pharmaceuticals can't be found, use the next best thing—foreign medications that are marked for your particular ailment. Try to explain your problem to the pharmacist, get his recommendation, then compare products. Look at the ingredients and go by the advice in this book; you won't go wrong.

For example, you're in France, your child has diaper rash and you didn't think to bring along the Desitin. Here's what to do.

Take the baby to the pharmacy with you if you think you'll have difficulty explaining the problem to the pharmacist. Let him look at the child so he knows what you are talking about.

He hands you a tube of Mitosyl, a product that is manufactured in France. Although you don't recognize the brand name, you'll certainly appreciate the ingredients: *huile de foie de poisson* 20 g (fish liver oil 20 gm), *oxyde de zinc 27 g* (zinc oxide 27 gm), and *butyl hydroxy anisol 0.02 g* (butyl alcohol 0.02 gm.) Since this product is quite similar to Desitin, it will probably work just as well. Buy it, it's good! (As a matter of fact, Mitosyl is highly recommended for burns, bruises, insect bites and stings, plus poison oak and ivy, in addition to diaper rash and prickly heat. It is just one of hundreds of fine products made and marketed outside the U.S..)

COMMENTS AND CAUTIONS
Throughout this book, I have discussed only nonprescription, over-the-counter products that can be purchased without the supervision of a doctor and, hopefully, used in a conscientious program of self-directed medical therapy. In this Afterword, I will make a few changes.

Recognizing the need for stronger drugs when the common ailments get out of hand, I thought it would be helpful to recommend a few prescription products that might come in handy while traveling.

If you intend to visit those places where diarrhea is legend (Mexico, Central America, South America, Asia) codeine or Lomotil should replace the weaker OTC antidiarrheal drugs. Your personal physician can write you a prescription, and you can have it filled before starting your journey. It might also be a good idea to take along a few Compazine suppositories for vomiting. The OTC products are okay, but when vomiting is severe, oral medications are hard to take, and a stronger drug in suppository form would be more appropriate.

For all the other common ailments that might occur while traveling, the OTC recommendations in this book should be sufficient. Often, they are just as effective as prescription items and, usually, they cost much less.

Bon voyage!

RECOMMENDED TRAVEL SUPPLIES

(For specific brand names of OTC products, refer to the appropriate pages.)

Antibiotic cream or ointment (pages 143-44)
Antidiarrhea medications (pages 168-72)
Antihistamine (pages 255-56)
Band-Aids, adhesive tape, gauze bandages
Decongestant medication (pages 87-98)
Extra eyeglasses
Individually packaged moistened paper towels
Laxative medication (pages 116-25)
Nausea and vomit-control medication (pages 277-78)
Mild pain relievers (pages 6-14)
Motion sickness pills (pages 277-78)
Nasal sprays (see topical decongestants, pages 84-87)
Safety pins
Water purification tablets (halazone)

Bibliography

P. B. Cason and W. McDermott; *Cecil and Loeb Textbook of Medicine,* 13th edition; W. B. Saunders, Philadelphia, Pa.; 1971.

W. F. Ganong; *Review of Medical Physiology,* 6th edition; Lange Medical Publications, Los Altos, Ca.; 1971.

A. C. Guyton; *Textbook of Medical Physiology,* 4th edition; W. B. Saunders, Philadelphia, Pa.; 1971.

Handbook of Non-Prescription Drugs, 5th edition; American Pharmaceutical Association, Washington, D.C.; 1977.

D. N. Holvey; *The Merck Manual of Diagnosis and Therapy,* 12th edition; Merck, Sharp, and Dohme Research Laboratories, Rahway, N.J.; 1972.

Physicians' Desk Reference, Medical Economics Company, Oradell, N.J., 1977.

Red Book 1977, Medical Economics Company, Oradell, N.J., 1977.

S. L. Robbins; *Pathological Basis of Disease,* 4th edition; W. B. Saunders, Philadelphia, Pa.; 1974.

M. M. Wintrobe et al.; *Harrison's Principles of Internal Medicine,* 7th edition; McGraw-Hill, New York, N.Y.; 1974.

Index

349